Contents

The Vaccines

Practical Information

Travel and Immunization

Foreword

Immunization against infectious disease is so effective and such an established part of medical practice that there is a danger that doctors and patients will take its success for granted. Yet there continue to be advances in the field with new and more effective vaccines for children, for at-risk groups and for the world traveller. One consequence is that immunization schedules have to be modified to ensure the greatest efficacy. Immunization has become a rapidly changing area of practice.

George Kassianos is a GP who has had a particular interest in immunization for many years. In this text, he builds on the success of the first edition with a clear presentation of the principles of immunization, detailed descriptions of the vaccines used and with practical guidance on their use. This book will be of immense help to doctors and nurses responsible for immunization programmes who are seeking practical guidance when planning for the needs of individual patients.

W. McN. Styles
Chairman of the Council
Royal College of General Practitioners

v

Preface

Immunization is one of the areas at the forefront of paediatric care in general practice. Effective and safe immunization, providing lasting immunity against infectious diseases, has made a major contribution to human welfare. Smallpox has been eradicated and, in countries with successful immunization programmes, we are witnessing virtual elimination of tetanus, diphtheria, poliomyelitis, pertussis, measles, mumps and rubella. The better the immunization programme, the greater the reduction in the morbidity and mortality of both bacterial and viral infectious diseases.

In most circumstances immunization, particularly of young children, is an elective procedure. The vaccines used to immunize children against infectious diseases are among the safest medicines available to GPs. It is, therefore, important to ascertain that no contraindications exist before any vaccination is carried out. To deny a child vaccination can be to deny that child health.

Part of the GP's work is confidently to promote the benefits of immunization. This has to be done in the face of both sporadic media scares and not only some hostility but also apathy among a minority of our patients.

Members of the primary care team involved in immunization should speak with one voice and give similar and consistent advice and information to parents. This book is intended to help the GP, health visitor and practice nurse to erect a united front in the fight for the total elimination of infectious diseases.

This second edition has been greatly revised and extended to include comprehensive advice on all immunizations performed in general practice.

I am very grateful to all those who have helped in the production of this book, especially to Nathalie Manners and Rebecca Huxley for all their hard work.

G.C. Kassianos

Abbreviations

AAFB	Acid and alcohol-fast bacterium
Ads	Adsorbed
AIDS	Acquired immune deficiency syndrome
Anti-HBc	Antibody to hepatitis B core antigen
Anti-HBe	Antibody to hepatitis B e antigen
Anti-HBs	Antibody to hepatitis B surface antigen
APV	Acellular pertussis vaccine
BCG	Bacillus Calmette-Guérin vaccine
BP	British Pharmacopoeia
CDSC	Communicable Diseases Surveillance Centres
CRS	Congenital rubella syndrome
DoH	Department of Health
DT	Diphtheria tetanus combined vaccine
DTP	Diphtheria tetanus pertussis combined vaccine
ELISA	Enzyme-linked immunoadsorbent assayed
eIPV	Enhanced potency inactivated poliomyelitis vaccine
HAV	Hepatitis A virus
HBV	Hepatitis B virus
HBeAg	Hepatitis B e antigen
HBIg	Hepatitis B immunoglobulin
HBsAg	Hepatitis B surface antigen
Hib	*Haemophilus influenzae* b vaccine
HIV	Human immunodeficiency virus
HNIG	Human normal immunoglobulin
HVZIG	Human varicella-zoster immunoglobulin
ID	Intradermal
Ig	Immunoglobulin
IM	Intramuscular
IPV	Inactivated poliomyelitis vaccine
IU	International unit
IV	Intravenous
MASTA	Medical Advisory Centre for Travellers Abroad
MMR	Measles mumps rubella combined vaccine
OP	Original pack

ABBREVIATIONS

OPCS	Office of Population Censuses and Surveys
OPV	Oral poliomyelitis vaccine
PHLS	Public Health Laboratory Services
SC	Subcutaneous
SSPE	Subacute sclerosing panencephalitis
UKCC	United Kingdom Central Council for Nurses, Midwives and Health Visitors
WHO	World Health Organization
VZV	Varicella zoster virus

Timescale of vaccine introduction in the UK

1938   Smallpox vaccination — the only routine immunization
Tetanus toxoid — for military personnel

1940   Diphtheria toxoid immunization (in some cities it began in 1937)

1950   BCG vaccination for health service staff and contacts of tuberculous patients

1953   BCG vaccination in general use
Pertussis vaccine (usually combined with diphtheria)

1956   Inactivated polio vaccine (Salk) — injectable

1956–1961 Tetanus toxoid routinely for children, initially in some areas as monovalent and nationally in 1961 as diphtheria/tetanus/pertussis (DTP)

1961   DTP combined vaccine

1962   Oral polio vaccine (Sabin)

1968   Measles vaccine

1970   Rubella vaccine for schoolgirls aged 11–13 years

1982   Hepatitis B plasma-derived vaccine

1987   Hepatitis B recombinant yeast vaccine

1988   Measles/mumps/rubella (MMR) combined vaccine

1989   Meningococcal A and C vaccine

1992   Hepatitis A vaccine
Haemophilus influenzae b vaccine
Oral and Typhim Vi typhoid vaccines

1994   Low-dose diphtheria and tetanus vaccine for adults and adolescents
Acellular monovalent pertussis vaccine

Notes

Current schedule of routine immunization for children in the UK

Age	Vaccine	Dose/route	Comment
2 months	Triple (DTP Ads*) Hib ‡ Polio	0.5 ml IM/SC 0.5 ml IM/SC 3 drops orally §	If pertussis vaccine is contraindicated, DT Ads† should be considered
3 months	Triple (DTP Ads) Hib Polio	0.5 ml IM/SC 0.5 ml IM/SC 3 drops orally	
4 months	Triple (DTP Ads) Hib Polio	0.5 ml IM/SC 0.5 ml IM/SC 3 drops orally	
12–15 months	MMR	0.5 ml IM/SC	1–15 years not previously vaccinated
4–5 years	DT Ads Polio	0.5 ml IM/SC 3 drops orally	Nursery or primary school entry
10–14 years	Rubella	0.5 ml IM/SC	Girls aged 10–14 not previously immunized or not wishing to have MMR. Seronegative women of childbearing age and seronegative male staff of antenatal clinics
10–14 years	BCG	0.1 ml ID	If tuberculin negative. At birth for babies in danger of contact with tuberculosis (0.05 ml)
15–19 years	Adsorbed diphtheria and tetanus vaccine for adults and adolescents Polio	0.5 ml IM/SC 3 drops orally	School-leavers

*DTP Ads: diphtheria, tetanus, pertussis adsorbed vaccine.
†DT Ads: diphtheria, tetanus adsorbed vaccine.
‡Hib: *Haemophilus influenzae* b vaccine (conjugated).
§Three drops or one monodose.

Notes

Viral and bacterial vaccines

	Viral vaccines	Bacterial vaccines
Live	Measles Mumps Rubella Oral poliomyelitis Yellow fever Varicella	BCG Oral typhoid
Inactivated	Influenza Hepatitis A Injectable poliomyelitis Rabies Tick-borne encephalitis Japanese B encephalitis	Pertussis Cholera Typhoid Plague
Toxoids		Diphtheria Tetanus
Bioengineered	Hepatitis B	
Polysaccharide extracts		*Haemophilus influenzae* b Meningoccocal A and C Pneumococcal Vi typhoid

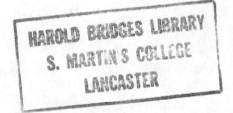

Notes

Special precautions for all vaccines

- All immunizations should be postponed if the patient is suffering from any acute febrile illness, particularly respiratory, until fully recovered. A minor infection without fever is not a reason for delaying immunization; this is particularly true for well babies who always seem snuffly.
- In general, it is not necessary to recommence a primary course of immunization however long a period has elapsed since the last dose was given. In infants whose basic course of DTP or poliomyelitis vaccine has been interrupted, a single dose later in infancy (or two doses where only the first dose of the basic course had been given) is adequate to establish immunity, regardless of the time elapsing between the initial and subsequent doses.
- Where possible an interval of at least 2 weeks should separate elective surgery from administering a vaccine.
- No immunization should be given to a site showing signs of skin infection.
- Vaccines must be stored under the conditions recommended by the manufacturers, usually at a refrigerator temperature of between +2 and +8°C (36–46°F). Do not freeze vaccines as this could cause deterioration of the product or breakage of the diluent container. Heat also causes deterioration of vaccines.
- Add the diluent slowly. Injecting with too much pressure will result in frothing with possible adverse effects on the vaccine efficacy.
- Multidose vials should be discarded after a vaccination session.
- Some vaccines contain traces of antibiotics. Severe sensitivity to a particular antibiotic means an anaphylactic reaction and not just a rash.
- Premature babies should have their first injection 2 months from the actual rather than expected date of birth.
- In adults avoid the left arm where possible as ischaemic heart pain radiating to the left upper limb may be considered by a patient as pain resulting from his or her recent vaccination.
- In the UK there is a popular belief that babies should not be taken to their local swimming pool until they have completed their first three

immunizations. This is yet another myth about immunization that needs to be dispelled.

● The site of vaccination is important. Injection of a vaccine into a buttock may be associated with a reduced antibody level production. The deltoid in adults and the anterolateral thigh in children are the preferred sites for most vaccinations.

Special precautions for live vaccines

● Live viral vaccines are inactivated by any pre-existing antibodies and, therefore, may be ineffective if given within a few weeks of administration of immunoglobulin or a blood transfusion.

● Live viral vaccines can also be inactivated if given to infants of mothers who at the time of pregnancy were immune (except oral poliovirus vaccine) — this is why the MMR vaccination is delayed until the child is over 1 year old.

● Reconstituted vaccines should be discarded if not used within the reconstituted life of the vaccine as recommended by the manufacturer, usually 1 h.

● A single injection of live viral vaccine produces long-term immunity and is not given more than once (except yellow fever for travel purposes). Oral poliovirus vaccine, however, contains three different components and is given more than once to ensure an adequate response to each component.

● Live virus vaccines that are not combined preparations, may be given simultaneously. If not given simultaneously an interval of at least 3 weeks should separate their administration. If a live virus vaccine is given soon after another live virus vaccine has been given, it is possible that the replication and the 'take' of the second vaccine would be interfered with by interferon or other inhibitory effects of the first vaccination. No live vaccine interferes with the activity of any dead vaccine.

● A 3-week interval is recommended between the administration of live virus vaccines and the giving of BCG (live bacterial vaccine) but may be given simultaneously and at a different site.

● With the exception of polio (see p. 39) and yellow fever (see p. 113), live vaccines should not be given within 3 months following the administration of human normal immunoglobulin (HNIG):

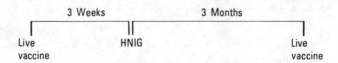

9

● Live vaccines should not be administered to persons whose ability to respond to infection is reduced for one reason or another. These vaccines should not be given to persons suffering from malignant disease, gammaglobulin deficiency or to those with impaired immune responsiveness, whether idiopathic or as a result of treatment with steroids, radiotherapy, cytotoxic drugs or other agents. Children with malignancy but off all treatment for more than 6 months may be immunized. Close contacts of immunodeficient children and adults must be immunized, particularly against measles and polio but not with oral polio vaccine (the inactivated, injectable vaccine is preferred).

● *An immunodeficient child* according to the Department of Health (DoH) is defined as follows:

(a) with serious conditions of the reticuloendothelial system (leukaemia, lymphomas, etc.);

(b) with primary immunodeficiency conditions — not human immunodeficiency virus (HIV) infection (see below);

(c) on doses of systemic steroids equivalent to 2 mg/kg per day or more of prednisolone, for at least 1 week within the preceding 3 months. Postpone vaccination until 3 months after stopping the steroid. A child on lower daily doses of systemic steroids for less than 2 weeks, or on lower doses on alternate-day regimens for longer periods, may be given live virus vaccines; and/or

(d) receiving chemotherapy. Postpone vaccination until at least 6 months after completion of chemotherapy.

● *An immunodeficient adult* is a patient with malignancy or primary immunodeficiency condition, or on chemotherapy or radiotherapy or receiving 60 mg or more of prednisolone daily.

● Give the vaccines 6 months after chemotherapy has finished or 3 months after treatment with systemic steroids has stopped. Use immunoglobulin in case of exposure to a virus.

● *Patients with HIV* (HIV positive) whether symptomatic or not, could be given all vaccines (MMR, DTP, typhoid, cholera, hepatitis B) but not BCG and yellow fever vaccines. Inactivated polio vaccine should be used instead of oral polio vaccine in HIV positive symptomatic patients.

● Live vaccines should not be administered to *pregnant women*, particularly early in pregnancy, because of possible harm to the fetus. However, where there is significant risk of exposure to such serious conditions as poliomyelitis or yellow fever, the importance of vaccination may outweigh the possible risk to the fetus.

● The parents of *children with a tendency to have convulsions* should be counselled on the management of any fever developing after immunization. Febrile convulsions may occur 5–10 days after measles immunization (or MMR) whereas they may take place in the first 72 h after pertussis immunization. Suggestions may include paracetamol, sponge with tepid water, give extra fluids, dress in thin clothing and place in a cool room. In high-risk children, an antipyretic drug may be suggested routinely for the first 72 h after immunization. Where the tendency is severe, the parents may be instructed on rectal diazepam administration.

● Report reactions to the Committee on Safety of Medicines (1 Nine Elms Lane, London SW8 5NQ, tel: 0171 273 3000) and also to the manufacturer (see p. 215).

Notes

Treating anaphylaxis

Although an anaphylactic reaction following vaccination is rare (118 cases reported between 1978 and 1989 — no deaths) any health-care personnel administering a vaccine should know what action to take on occurrence.

Anaphylactic reaction may occur within seconds or minutes of injection. The patient suddenly sweats profusely and looses consciousness. Alternatively, the onset may be gradual with urticaria, angio-oedema (hoarseness, stridor, dyspnoea), pallor and collapse.

A strong central pulse (carotid or femoral) is more likely to indicate a simple faint (common in older children and adults) whilst a weak central pulse may indicate anaphylaxis in which case the following instructions should be followed:

- place the patient in the left lateral ('recovery') position;
- insert airway (if unconscious);
- administer oxygen if available;
- administer adrenaline 1 : 1000 (1 mg/ml) by deep IM injection and repeat in 10 min if required, up to a maximum of three doses, in a dose of 0.01 ml/kg bodyweight or in the doses listed in Table 1;
- in adults hydrocortisone 100 mg or chlorpheniramine maleate (Piriton) 10–20 mg IV may be given;
- children may also need to receive hydrocortisone IV (up to 1 year, 25 mg; 1–5 years, 50 mg; 6–12 years, 100 mg);

Table 1 Recommended doses of adrenaline in the treatment of anaphylaxis

Adrenaline 1 : 1000 (1 mg/ml)	Dosage (ml)
3–5 months	0.05
6–11 months	0.75
1 year	0.1
2 years	0.2
3–4 years	0.3
5 years	0.4
6–10 years	0.5
Older children and adults	0.5–1

- it is recommended that all cases of anaphylaxis are admitted to hospital for observation;
- report the reaction to the Committee on Safety of Medicines and if possible to the manufacturer;
- the adrenaline injection solution deteriorates, particularly when exposed to light; replace ampoules annually (my own policy is to do this every Christmas) or at expiry date, whichever is earlier, and follow manufacturer's instructions.

THE VACCINES

Diphtheria/tetanus/pertussis (DTP) combined and diphtheria/tetanus (DT) combined

Contraindications to vaccination
Those of the monovalent vaccine are described under diphtheria vaccine (p. 21), tetanus vaccine (p. 25) and pertussis vaccine (p. 29).

Possible side and adverse effects

Local reactions
Swelling and redness at the site of injection can appear within the first 48–72 h, and may last up to 1–2 weeks. A painless lump can appear under the skin within 1 week, especially when the injection was not given deep enough. It may persist for several weeks.

General reactions
The reader is referred to the section on general reactions of the monovalent vaccines (pp. 21, 25, 30). A brief summary is provided of a report from the Institute of Medicine (USA) on DTP vaccine-related adverse events (*JAMA* 1992; 267: 3):

- *Acute encephalopathy:* the range of excess risk of acute encephalopathy following DTP immunization is consistent with that estimated for the British National Encephalopathy Study: 0.0–10.5 per million immunizations;
- *Shock and 'unusual shock-like state':* the evidence did not provide for reliable estimates of excess risk following DTP immunization. Reported incidence in literature varies from 3.5 to 291 cases per 100 000 immunizations;
- *Anaphylaxis:* in the absence of formal studies of incidence, rates of anaphylaxis are estimated to be approximately two cases per 100 000 injections of DTP (six cases per 100 000 children given three doses of DTP);
- *Protracted, inconsolable crying:* incidence rates are estimated to range from 0.1 to 6% of recipients of a DTP injection and vary with type and dose of vaccine and with immunization site.

The vaccine

● Adsorbed DTP vaccine is an aqueous suspension containing a mixture of purified diphtheria and tetanus toxoids and killed *Bordetella pertussis* organisms, adsorbed onto aluminium hydroxide. Thiomersal is added as a preservative. Each 0.5 ml dose has a potency of not less than 30 IU of diphtheria toxoid, not less than 60 IU of tetanus toxoid and not less than 4 IU of *Bordetella pertussis* cells.

● Adsorbed DT vaccine is similar to DTP but without the pertussis component and with a reduced content (not less than 40 IU) of tetanus toxoid. It can only be used in the under 10 year olds.

● Adsorbed DT Vaccine for Adults and Adolescents BP (Table 3) has been available in the UK since the summer of 1994. It contains not less than 4 IU of diphtheria toxoid and not less than 40 IU of tetanus toxoid, both adsorbed onto aluminium hydroxide with thiomersal added as a preservative. It is available for the immunization of adults and children over the age of 10 years.

● The triple adsorbed DTP vaccine is recommended for the primary course of infants from 2 months of age. The course consists of three doses with an interval of 1 month between each dose. Where the pertussis component is to be omitted, adsorbed DT is used instead. Each dose is 0.5 ml and is given by IM or deep SC injection. The container should be shaken before withdrawing the vaccine suspension.

Table 2 UK schedule of DTP immunization

Vaccine	2 months	3 months	4 months	4–5 years	15–19 years
Adsorbed DTP	0.5 ml	0.5 ml	0.5 ml	—	—
Adsorbed DT (only if pertussis is to be omitted)	0.5 ml	0.5 ml	0.5 ml	0.5 ml (all children)	—
Adsorbed DT Vaccine for Adults and Adolescents BP	—	—	—	—	0.5 ml

Table 3 Administration specifications for adsorbed DT Vaccine for Adults and Adolescents BP

Dose (ml)	Route	Primary immunization	Boosters
0.5	IM/SC	Three doses at monthly intervals (unimmunized adults only)	Every 10 or more years for those at risk, e.g. travellers

- A booster dose of adsorbed DT (pertussis omitted) is given at the age of 4–5 years, at school entry.
- DTP and DT should not be used in children over the age of 10 years.
- Over the age of 10 years, children used to receive a booster of monovalent adsorbed tetanus vaccine at school-leaving age (15–19 years). As from the autumn of 1994, school-leavers have received a booster of the Adsorbed DT Vaccine for Adults and Adolescents BP.
- If the primary course of DTP or DT is started later than 2 months of age (in the under 10 year olds), the booster dose of DT should be given 3 years later. Although a minimum of 5 years is normally recommended between tetanus boosters, there is no evidence that giving the booster a year or two early is associated with any increased risk of a severe reaction.
- Immunization with three doses of triple vaccine (DTP) at monthly intervals completed before 6 months of age probably provides adequate protection against diphtheria, tetanus and whooping cough which will persist until the age of the preschool booster (Ramsay et al., BMJ 1991; 302: 1489–91). A booster dose of DTP at 18 months and pertussis at 4–5 years is not recommended in the UK, while children in the USA receive boosters of DTP at 18 months and 4–6 years. Long-term follow-up of antibody concentrations in infants immunized on accelerated schedules introduced in 1990 are necessary to determine whether the British immunization policy should change.
- A future policy may be the administration of a combined DTP/Hib vaccine. Studies show such a combined vaccine elicits a greater immune response than the two vaccines given separately, although there is also a higher incidence of local reactions (JAMA 1992; 268 (24)).
- From the summer of 1994, the Adsorbed DT Vaccine for Adults and Adolescents BP became available. This vaccine is suitable for:
  (a) immunization of children over 10 years of age if primary immunization and/or reinforcing dose were not previously given;
  (b) to booster the immunity of school-leavers as part of the UK schedule of routine immunization for children;
  (c) for the primary immunization of unvaccinated adults;
  (d) for boosters for adults at risk, e.g. those travelling to endemic areas. The dose is 0.5 ml IM or SC.

Vaccine availability

● Trivax-AD (adsorbed DTP vaccine), Evans Medical Ltd, available in 0.5 and 5 ml ampoules.

● Adsorbed DTP vaccine, Merieux UK Ltd, available in prefilled syringes of 0.5 ml.

● Adsorbed DT Vaccine BP, available from both manufacturers listed above.

● All childhood immunization vaccines are distributed by Farillon Ltd free to GPs, on behalf of the DoH.

● Diftavax Adsorbed DT Vaccine for Adults and Adolescents BP, Merieux UK Ltd, available as a single-dose, 0.5 ml vaccine for primary immunization or boosters for adults. For booster of school-leavers, the vaccine is distributed free of charge to GPs, by Farillon, on behalf of the DoH, in packs of 5 × 0.5 ml ampoules. They should be ordered directly from Farillon Ltd.

Storage. Between +2 and +8°C. *Do not freeze.* Protect from light. Discard any partly used vaccine in multidose containers at the end of a vaccination session.

Diphtheria

Contraindications to vaccination
- Acute febrile illness.
- Severe reaction such as a neurological or anaphylactic reaction to an earlier diphtheria immunization.
- Severe hypersensitivity to aluminium and/or thiomersal.
- Pregnancy — there are no data on the use of diphtheria vaccine in pregnancy. Do not use in pregnancy unless the mother is at increased risk.

Possible side and adverse effects

Local reactions
- Swelling, redness and pain.
- A small painless nodule may form at the injection site but usually disappears without sequelae.

General reactions
- Transient fever, headaches, malaise, rarely urticaria, pallor and dyspnoea.
- Neurological reactions very rarely occur.

The vaccine
- The Adsorbed Diphtheria Vaccine BP is a suspension of highly purified toxoid from the exotoxin of *Corynebacterium diphtheriae*, adsorbed onto hydrated aluminium phosphate. Thiomersal is added as a preservative. The immunizing potency of each 0.5 ml dose is not less than 30 IU (the old system of flocculation units Lf merely expressed the quantity of toxoid present). (A low-dose diphtheria vaccine for adults is also available.)
- *Indications:* for active immunization against diphtheria of children under the age of 10, where a combined DTP or DT vaccine was not used. Three doses of 0.5 ml are given 1 month apart, by IM or deep SC injection. Children receiving their primary course in infancy should receive a reinforcing dose of 0.5 ml at about 5 years of age.

- An interrupted primary course should not be repeated but continued.
- Diphtheria vaccine is available in the following combinations:
  (a) adsorbed diphtheria vaccine;
  (b) adsorbed low-dose diphtheria vaccine for adults;
  (c) adsorbed DTP vaccine;
  (d) adsorbed DT vaccine;
  (e) adsorbed DT Vaccine for Adults and Adolescents BP.
- For primary immunization or boosters of children over the age of 10 years and adults: when a monovalent diphtheria vaccine is necessary the Adsorbed Low-Dose Diphtheria Vaccine for Adults BP should be used. The dose is 0.5 ml both for boosters and the primary immunization course, which consists of three doses of the vaccine by deep SC or IM injection at intervals of 1 month.
- Material for Schick testing is no longer available in the UK.
- The 1993 outbreak of diphtheria in the Russian Federation (over 15 000 cases in 1993) and the Ukraine caused in the UK a shortage of low-dose single antigen diphtheria vaccine for adults. The DoH advises diphtheria immunization of travellers at risk, i.e. those who will have close contact with the local population, such as health workers and teachers intending to work in the Russian Federation or Ukraine, travellers staying for more than 1 month, and people who are likely to share accommodation overnight or have kissing or sexual contact with local people. Such unvaccinated travellers should receive a full primary course of diphtheria vaccine. To overcome the shortage of low-dose diphtheria vaccine the DoH suggested the use of combined tetanus toxoid/low-dose diphtheria (Diftavax) vaccine, that is available from Merieux UK Ltd. The diphtheria content in this vaccine has been reduced to about one-tenth of its 'original' value, while that of the tetanus toxoid remains the same (each single dose is 0.5 ml of the vaccine). This vaccine was licensed in the summer of 1994 (see pp. 18, 19, 20).
- Unimmunized contacts of a case of diphtheria should be immunized and should receive a prophylactic course of erythromycin.
- HIV infected children may be immunized against diphtheria.
- Diphtheria antitoxin is only used in suspected cases of diphtheria infection.
- The level of diphtheria antitoxin titres necessary for protection is 0.01 IU/ml.
- Immunity is over 10 years.

• Control of diphtheria depends on widespread acceptance of immunization in order to create herd and individual immunity. Vaccine-induced immunity tends to wane. With a large vaccine uptake as in the UK (94% of 1 year olds in 1993) there is decreased frequency of exposure to the organism and, therefore, decreased maintenance of immunity secondary to community contact. Many adults are susceptible to diphtheria — in the mid-1980s this was estimated at 30% of young adults and over 40% of the older groups. The USA also face a similar problem. There is, therefore, a case for recommending regular booster injections of diphtheria toxoid every 10 years after completion of the primary immunization. As yet, this recommendation has not been put forward by the DoH. On the other hand, the DoH is now recommending including diphtheria when performing the school-leavers' booster (low-dose DT Vaccine for Adults and Adolescents BP, see pp. 18, 19, 20). This vaccine may be used for primary immunization of the unvaccinated patient, or as a booster of previously immunized adults when travelling to at-risk areas.

Vaccine availability
• Adsorbed low-dose diphtheria vaccine for adults, Regent Labs Ltd, available in 5 ml vials and 0.5 ampoules.
• Adsorbed Diphtheria Vaccine BP, Evans Medical Ltd, available in 0.5 ml ampoules.

Storage. Between +2 and +8°C. *Do not freeze.* Protect from light.

Diphtheria infection
This is caused by *Corynebacterium diphtheriae*, a Gram-positive club-shaped rod which produces a membrane in the throat of infected patients. It is an acute infection of the upper respiratory tract and occasionally it involves the skin too. Life-threatening complications of diphtheria include obstructive laryngotracheitis, myocarditis, thrombocytopenia, paralysis of the vocal cords, and ascending paralysis similar to that of Guillain–Barré syndrome.

There are two strains of the bacterium: one toxigenic and the other non-toxigenic. The former is responsible for the classical manifestations of the disease. Humans are the only reservoir of the bacterium. Transmission results from intimate contact with a patient or carrier and by droplet infection. The incubation period is 2–5 days and the infectivity period in untreated persons lasts for 2–4 weeks. Occasionally carriers can shed the organism for several months. The organism is sensitive to erythromycin which is also given to contacts.

Diptheria vaccine was introduced in the UK in 1940. It has had a dramatic effect on the incidence of diphtheria and has virtually eliminated the disease in the UK. Nonetheless, sporadic cases do occur although most of them are imported.

Finally, it is important to remember that although diphtheria is most severe in unimmunized or inadequately immunized persons, it can also infect people who have been immunized in the past according to the schedule recommended by the DoH.

Table 4 Rates of diphtheria infection in the UK

Period	Notifications	Deaths
1940	46 281	6
1957	37	0
1986–1992	21	0

Tetanus

Contraindications to vaccination
- Acute febrile illness, unless the patient has a tetanus-prone wound in which case the vaccine is indicated.
- Severe local reaction (swelling and redness affecting most of the circumference of the limb injected) and general reaction (fever > 39.5°C within 48 h of injection, laryngeal oedema, bronchospasm, peripheral neuropathy, anaphylaxis) to a previously administered dose of the vaccine.
- Severe hypersensitivity to aluminium and thiomersal (except Clostet, Evans Medical Ltd as it does not contain thiomersal).
- During the first year after a primary course or a booster (a hypersensitivity reaction may be provoked).
- May be used in pregnancy only if absolutely necessary.

Possible side and adverse effects

Local reactions
Swelling, redness and pain may develop up to 10 days after injection. Not deep enough injection may result in a persistent nodule at the site of injection.

General reactions
Pyrexia, headaches, malaise and myalgia. Urticaria and acute anaphylactic reaction occasionally occur. Peripheral neuropathy is rare.

The vaccine
- Adsorbed tetanus vaccine is a suspension of purified tetanus toxoid, adsorbed onto aluminium. Each 0.5 ml dose has an immunizing potency of not less than 40 IU. It stimulates the production of antitoxin which provides immunity against the effects of the tetanus toxin.
- The available adsorbed tetanus vaccines are monovalent, or combined with diphtheria (DT), or with diphtheria and pertussis (DTP).
- Tetanus vaccine in simple solution (plain) has also been available but

it is less immunogenic than the adsorbed vaccine and has no advantage in terms of reaction rates. It is no longer available in the UK since July 1994.

Administration

• The dose for all ages is 0.5 ml, given by deep SC or IM injection.

• Children under the age of 10 years should receive DTP (or DT if pertussis is contraindicated) at the age of 2, 3 and 4 months and a DT booster prior to school entry. A second booster is given before leaving secondary school with low-dose diphtheria combined with tetanus vaccine — see DTP and DT vaccines, pp. 18, 19, 20.

• Adults and children over 10 years that have not previously been immunized should be immunized according to the schedule outlined in Table 5.

• If a course is interrupted, it should just be continued and not restarted.

• A wound or burn is considered tetanus-prone if (a) it is a puncture-type wound; (b) it has come in contact with soil or manure; (c) clinical evidence of sepsis is present; or (d) surgical treatment of the wound or burn has been delayed for more than 6 h. In the event of such a wound occurring on a patient who has not fully completed the primary course, this should be completed; if the last booster was given 10 or more years ago, another booster should be given; if the patient is unimmunized or uncertain, a full three-dose course should be given. In all the above cases a dose of antitetanus immunoglobulin should be given IM and at a different site than the vaccine, at the following doses (adults and children):

    (a) within 24 h from the injury, 250 IU (1 ml ampoule); or

    (b) over 24 h from the injury, 500 IU.

• In the event of the antitetanus immunoglobulin being used for

Table 5 Immunization schedule for tetanus in the UK for adults and children over 10 years

Dose (ml)	Route	Primary immunization course	Boosters
0.5	Deep SC or IM	0, 1 month, 2 months (three doses)	Every 10 years for two doses*

* Further 10-yearly boosters are not recommended in the UK, other than at the time of injury or travel to at-risk areas.

treatment of tetanus, the dose is 30–300 IU (average 150 IU) per kilogram of bodyweight given IM.

- HIV infected children and adults should be considered for tetanus immunization.
- Tetanus vaccine became available for use with armed forces personnel in 1938. Male patients who were in the British forces during the Second World War were fully immunized. A considerable number of male teenagers would have received tetanus immunization during their national service in the immediate years following the war. While many authorities had provided vaccination previously, it was not until 1961 that childhood immunization against tetanus was recommended nationally by the DoH. Tetanus immunization was also offered to members of groups who were at particular risk, e.g. farm workers.
- Unlike diphtheria, tetanus control does not depend on herd immunity since *Clostridium tetani* is widely distributed in soil and animal excreta. The object of immunization is to protect each individual directly.
- Statistics show that the highest risk groups are elderly, particularly women. Of all tetanus cases notified between 1985 and 1991, 53% were people over the age of 65. Serological studies in the USA indicate that at least 40% of people over the age of 60 do not have a protective serum level of antitoxin. Similarly, 11% of adults aged 18–39 years lack protective levels of antitoxin. Inadequate immunity may result from failure to receive primary immunization or to have boosters at the recommended intervals (10-yearly boosters are recommended in the USA).

Vaccine availability
- CLoSTET Adsorbed Tetanus Vaccine, Evans Medical Ltd.
- Tetavax, Merieux UK Ltd.
- Servier Adsorbed Tetanus Vaccine, Servier Laboratories Ltd.
All available in single-dose 0.5 ml prefilled syringes.

Storage. Between +2 and +8°C. *Do not freeze.* Protect from light.

Antitetanus immunoglobulin availability
- Bio Products Laboratory.
- Regional blood transfusion centres.

Storage. Between +2 and +8°C. *Do not freeze.*

Tetanus infection

It is caused by *Clostridium tetani*, a Gram-positive bacillus that grows under anaerobic conditions. Soil is its natural habitat. Its spores can also be found in the faeces of domestic animals and even in human faeces. It is distributed worldwide.

Clostridium tetani produces two toxins: tetanospasmin and tetano-lysin. Only the former is significant as it reaches the spinal cord and brain via blood and peripheral nerves. It increases reflex excitability in motor neurones by blocking the function of inhibitory neurones. It can affect the medullary centres and can pass along sympathetic fibres leading to overactivity of the sympathetic nervous system too.

The incubation period is between 4 and 21 days. The onset is gradual and progresses to rigidity and severe muscular spasms which can lead to respiratory failure.

Neonatal tetanus due to infection of the baby's umbilical stump is a common cause of neonatal mortality in many countries in Africa and Asia. It is relatively rare in Europe although cases still occur. It kills half a million babies every year and in some countries it accounts for half of neonatal mortality. It is preventable by immunizing women with tetanus toxoid, by clean delivery and post-delivery care. In 1989 the World Health Organization (WHO) adopted the goal of eliminating neonatal tetanus from the world by 1995. As a result the proportion of women in developing countries having at least two doses of tetanus toxoid rose from 18% in 1986 to 56% in 1990.

Tetanus is a rare disease in the UK. Nonetheless, sporadic cases (including deaths) do occur, mainly among elderly people who are at greatest risk. Between 1984 and 1991, 116 cases were notified to Communicable Diseases Surveillance Centres (CDSC) in England and Wales, and a further 10 cases in 1992. There was one death in 1990, three in 1991 and one in 1992 attributed to tetanus infection.

Pertussis

Contraindications to vaccination
- Acute febrile illness.
- Severe hypersensitivity to aluminium and thiomersal.
- Severe local (extensive redness and hard swelling involving much of the circumference of the limb at the injection site) or general reaction (fever > 39.5°C within 48 h of vaccination, prolonged unresponsiveness, prolonged inconsolable or high-pitched screaming for more than 4 h, convulsions or encephalopathy occurring within 72 h of vaccination, or any of the following: anaphylaxis, bronchospasm, laryngeal oedema, generalized collapse) to a previous pertussis or pertussis-containing vaccine.
- Unstable or evolving neurological problem — defer until the condition is stable (administration of pertussis vaccine may coincide with or hasten the recognition of inevitable manifestations of the progressive disorder, with resulting confusion about causation, e.g. uncontrolled epilepsy, infantile spasms, progressive encephalopathy).
- Pregnancy, unless a young mother is at great risk in which case her risk may outweigh the theoretical risk to the fetus.

Children with a problem history
- The child with immediate family (parents and siblings) history of epilepsy: although the risk of seizures in such children is increased, these are usually febrile in origin and have a generally benign outcome. Subsequent developmental progress of these children has not been found to have been impaired. Immunize and advise on management of fever (see p. 11).
- The child with personal history of epilepsy: there is an increased risk of convulsions after pertussis immunization, and this is probably simply a reflection of the pyrogenic nature of pertussis cellular vaccine. In the UK, pertussis vaccine is rarely given to children when they are of an age to have a confirmed diagnosis of epilepsy. Immunize and advise on management of fever. Some parents may have to be supplied and instructed on the use of rectal diazepam, to use if convulsions occur, while awaiting the arrival of the GP.

• The child with personal or family history of febrile convulsions: immunize but advise on management of fever and appropriate medical care in the event of a seizure.

• The child with stable neurological conditions: these patients should be immunized (examples include children with cerebral palsy or spina bifida).

• In advising parents of children with a problem history, the GP should inform them of the risks and benefits of pertussis immunization and should give advice on how to manage the child's fever or seizure should it occur. An unvaccinated child will remain susceptible to pertussis infection. If in doubt, seek advice from the hospital or community paediatrician.

Possible side and adverse effects
Adverse effects (especially local reactions and pyrexia) are fewer when the new British accelerated schedule of immunization (starting at 2 months of age) is used compared with the extended schedules which used to go into the second half of the first year of life, when febrile convulsions without immunizations are more common.

Local reactions
Swelling, redness and pain. A small painless nodule may form at the injection site but usually disappears without sequelae.

General reactions
• Fever, crying, screaming and irritability may occur after pertussis vaccination and also when pertussis is omitted and DT vaccine only is given. Inconsolable screaming or crying (sometimes high-pitched) may last over 3 h and occur within the first 48 h.

• Transient urticarial rashes: unless appearing within minutes of vaccination are unlikely to be anaphylactic in origin.

• Seizures occurring within 48 h of administration of pertussis vaccine are rare (incidence put at 1 in 2000–10 000). They occur usually in febrile children, are brief, generalized and self-limiting (usually febrile convulsions). Predisposing factors are personal and/or family history of convulsions.

• Collapse can occur rarely. These children's developmental progress has been found subsequently to be normal.

• Severe anaphylactic reactions are very rare.

● Encephalopathy, permanent neurological disability (brain damage) and even death have in the past been considered as rare sequelae of pertussis immunization. Such adverse events and illnesses can occur in immunized and unimmunized children from a variety of causes, particularly in the first year of life. As there is no specific test, determination of whether pertussis vaccine is the cause is not possible.

● Public and professional anxiety about the safety of pertussis vaccine resulted from the UK National Childhood Encephalopathy Study contacted between 1976 and 1979. This study, at the time, indicated that the risk of encephalopathy was 1 in 140 000 doses of pertussis vaccine and that the risk of permanent brain damage was 1 in 330 000. Further and later analysis of these data indicated that the above encephalopathy rate was developed by, among others, adding in a number of children with febrile convulsions, which are not usually associated with permanent sequelae. If those subjects are excluded, the remaining numbers are too small to show conclusively whether or not the vaccine can cause such adverse effects. The conclusion is, therefore, that although the data do not prove pertussis vaccine can never cause encephalopathy/brain damage, nonetheless they do indicate that if it does so, such occurrences must be exceedingly rare. There are no specific tests available to identify cases which may have been caused by pertussis vaccine. The benefits of pertussis vaccine outweigh the risks.

● Three recent American studies have re-examined the risks of febrile seizures and other neurological events after immunization with pertussis-containing vaccines (*JAMA* 1990; 263: 1641–5). The total number of subjects was 230 000 with more than 700 000 immunizations. There were no proven vaccine-induced permanent central nervous system injuries. J. Cherry in an editorial (*JAMA* 1990; 263: 1679–80) commenting on these studies indicated that 'the myth of encephalopathy should end'.

● GPs counselling parents about pertussis immunization may wish to have in mind the following review by Dr G.S. Golden, an American paediatric neurologist (Pertussis vaccine and injury to brain, *J Paediatr* 1990; 116: 854–61). His conclusions are as follows:

(a) population studies, particularly the UK National Childhood Encephalopathy Study, do not provide evidence of permanent neurological sequelae resulting from pertussis vaccine;

(b) there is no convincing evidence that children with a personal history of neurological disease, or family history of convulsions, will deteriorate more rapidly if they receive triple vaccine, although caution is usually advised;

(c) pertussis vaccine does not cause epilepsy, although about 1 in 10 000 children will have a febrile seizure;

(d) therre is no convincing evidence linking pertussis vaccine with infantile spasms;

(e) there is no convincing evidence of a casual link between pertussis immunization and sudden infant death syndrome (cot death);

(f) in cases where pertussis vaccine has been blamed for causing neurological damage, there are no specific neuropathological findings.

The vaccine

● Pertussis vaccine is a suspension of inactivated *Bordetella pertussis* and is usually given as part of the triple vaccine combined with diphtheria and tetanus vaccines.

● A monovalent whole-cell pertussis vaccine is available in the U K from Merieux U K Ltd, on a 'named patient' basis. It is the same pertussis vaccine that is incorporated in Merieux's D T P.

● No acellular pertussis-containing D T P vaccine is licensed in the U K (1994). Two acellular D T P vaccines are licensed in the U S A for use as an 18-month and preschool booster after data showed similar immunogenicity and reduced reactogenicity relative to whole-cell D T P vaccine.

● As yet, the U K has not licensed an acellular pertussis-containing D T P vaccine and will probably not be doing so until the results of a large Swedish trial are known. The current whole-cell pertussis-containing vaccine is effective and has an established safety record. The introduction of the accelerated immunization schedule in the U K (first triple at 2 months of age) has been associated with fewer minor reactions such as fever, further decline in disease incidence and deaths and an improvement in vaccine uptake. Therefore, the case for replacing the existing whole-cell D T P vaccine with acellular preparations needs to be convincing and in particular it requires evidence of better immunogenicity, reduced reactogenicity and potentially better vaccine uptake.

Administration

For administration of combined D T P vaccine, see p. 18.

● Pertussis monovalent vaccine is indicated for children when the pertussis component has been omitted from earlier immunizations. The full primary course should be given to children who have received previously a full course of D T. If the primary course was not completed, the D T P should be used to complete it and pertussis immunization

Table 6 Administration specifications for cellular pertussis monovalent vaccine ('named patient' basis)

Dose (ml)	Route	Primary course	Boosters
0.5	Deep SC or IM injection	Three doses at monthly intervals	None

should be completed with monovalent pertussis vaccine, always allowing 1 month between each injection.

● No boosters are recommended in the UK. Vaccination against pertussis and *Haemophilus influenzae* b are the only immunizations in infancy in the UK that are not reinforced when children first attend school.

● There is no upper age limit, therefore consider immunization of older children who have missed their pertussis vaccinations.

● If the primary course is interrupted, it should be resumed from where it was stopped and not repeated.

● It is not contraindicated for HIV positive individuals.

● If a febrile convulsion occurs after a dose of pertussis or pertussis-containing vaccine, the GP is advised to seek the advice of the hospital or community paediatrician before considering further vaccinations.

● An increased incidence of reactions may occur due to failure to shake the container to resuspend the vaccine before withdrawing the dose, inadvertent intravenous injection, or overrapid injection.

● An inadequately immunized 1-year-old child has a 1 in 6 chance of developing pertussis before the age of 10.

● The estimated efficacy of the vaccine is in excess of 80% after a full primary course (three doses).

● Vaccine-induced immunity persists for at least 3 years, and diminishes thereafter. Several years after vaccination, the efficacy is about 50%. No reinforcing doses are as yet recommended in the UK while American children receive two further reinforcing doses, one at 18 months and another around 5 years (as DTP).

● Pertussis infection in those immunized is usually mild.

Vaccine availability

Monovalent Pertussis Vaccine, Merieux UK Ltd, on a 'named patient' basis.

Storage. Between +2 and +8°C. *Do not freeze.* Shake before use.

Acellular monovalent pertussis vaccine

Contraindications to vaccination
● Acute febrile illness.
● Severe localized or generalized reaction to a preceeding dose of the acellular pertussis vaccine.
● Severe generalized reaction to a previously administered dose of the whole-cell pertussis vaccine.
● Any neurological condition in which there are changing developmental or neurological findings.
● Pregnancy, unless a young mother is at great risk.
A severe local reaction to the whole-cell pertussis-containing vaccine is not necessarily a contraindication to the acellular pertussis vaccine (APV), as the likelihood of such a reaction after APV is small.

Possible side and adverse effects
The APV is expected to be less reactogenic than the cellular pertussis vaccine and it will need to be evaluated in the UK under the new arrangements for its introduction (see below). Report all suspected side and adverse effects to the Committee on Safety of Medicines.

The vaccine
Single-antigen acellular pertussis vaccine adsorbed is an unlicensed product, being made available by the DoH under Crown Immunity (the Medicines Act 1968). It is available to doctors on a 'named patient' basis.

The acellular monovalent pertussis vaccine is already licensed in Germany as a monovalent product and in the USA as part of the trivalent DTP vaccine used for the 18-month and preschool boosters. Acellular pertussis vaccines have been in routine use for some time now in Japan.

Administration
● *Indications:* For children who have not received or partially completed their pertussis immunization; for babies whose parents refuse to allow vaccination with the existing whole-cell pertussis-containing DTP vaccine.
● APV should not be used as an alternative to the existing whole-cell pertussis-containing vaccine (combined with diphtheria and tetanus) as there is still no conclusive evidence of protective efficacy for APV.

Table 7 Administration specifications for acellular pertussis monovalent vaccine ('named patient' basis)

Dose (ml)	Route	Primary course	Boosters
0.5	IM or deep SC	Three injections at monthly intervals	None

● A primary course of immunization started with whole-cell vaccine can be completed with APV. If interrupted, there is no need to recommence the primary course and it should be completed.

● Members of the primary health-care team should promote the existing trivalent DTP vaccine and should counsel worried parents. Any baby whose pertussis immunization is delayed in the first years of life is in danger of infection. The APV should only be suggested as a last resort.

Vaccine availability

Monovalent acellular pertussis adsorbed vaccine is imported by Lederle Laboratories and distributed free of charge on behalf of the DoH by Farillon Ltd. Orders for the vaccine should be placed direct to Farillon Ltd, and should be accompanied by the patient's name. Available in single-dose 0.5 ml vials.

Storage. Between + 2 and + 8°C. *Do not freeze.*

Pertussis infection

Pertussis is caused by *Bordetella pertussis*, a small aerobic Gram-negative pleomorphic bacillus. Some cases are also attributed to *Bordetella parapertussis*. The bacillus adheres to the cilia of human respiratory tract epithelial cells where it multiplies and releases toxic substances.

Humans are the only known reservoir. It is transmitted by aerosol droplets from the respiratory tract of an infected patient. The incubation period is 1–3 weeks, usually 7–10 days.

The disease affects any age, but especially infants. It begins with mild upper respiratory tract symptoms and cough (catarrhal stage) when the patient is most infectious. Within 7–10 days the cough progresses to severe paroxysms (paroxysmal stage) that lasts usually about 1–2 months, followed by a decrease in symptoms (convalescent stage).

The characteristic whoop, when present (may be absent in young infants), is due to an inspiratory attempt to breathe in after the child is out of breath in a coughing spasm. It is more severe at night when the child can sound as if he or she is choking. During these spasmic periods apnoea can occur. In the attempt to clear the thick mucous the child with whooping cough vomits. There is little fever. The duration of the illness is 6–12 weeks and in spite of the above symptoms the child can appear well most of the time.

Complications that can arise are weight loss because of vomiting, bronchopneumonia, encephalopathy, seizures, permanent brain damage and death. The younger the child, the more common the complications.

Treatment with erythromycin decreases the likelihood of infection. The infected children usually become culture negative within 6 days and most will not relapse if the treatment course is continued for 14 days.

Pertussis morbidity and mortality are strongly correlated with socioeconomic conditions. It is a major public health problem, particularly for poor, malnourished infants in whom the mortality rates are far higher than among infants in developed countries. In the developing world the mortality rate is as high as 1 in 100 cases. More than 500 000 deaths worldwide are attributed to pertussis infection with probably over 60 000 000 cases of pertussis occurring every year. Countries with high immunization rates among infants have seen the virtual elimination of the disease.

In the U K the pertussis vaccine was introduced in 1953 and was soon to have a dramatic effect on the number of cases notified. But a few cases of alleged neurological damage associated with pertussis immunization were widely publicised by the media in the 1970s. Among the medical profession there was also disagreement especially after the publication of the paper 'Neurological complications of pertussis inoculation' by Kulenkampff *et al.* (*Arch Dis Child* 1974; 49: 46–9). Doctors started inventing contraindications (see Table 8) and the public lost its confidence in the vaccine. This resulted in a huge drop of vaccine acceptance from 80 to 30%. Pertussis infection became widespread with numbers of cases notified matching the pre-vaccine era, and deaths rising. These events provided the clearest evidence that the benefits of pertussis immunization outweighed the possible risks associated with it. Once the public's (and doctors') confidence was restored in the late 1980s, the rate of notifications and deaths again dropped dramatically. The restored high uptake of the vaccine has also seen the disappearance of the characteristic 2-year peaks and troughs (Table 9).

Table 8 The 1970s pertussis contraindications myths

Asthma, eczema, hayfever
Prematurity
Low attained weight
Breast feeding
Antibiotic treatment
Congenital heart disease
Chronic lung disease
Cerebral palsy and other neurological conditions
Chromosomal abnormalities
Topical or inhaled steroids
Pregnancy in mother
Family history of convulsions in distant relatives
Family history of immunization reaction
Previous mumps, measles or rubella infection
Jaundice after birth
'Snuffles'

Table 9 Benefits of pertussis immunization (England and Wales)

Year	Immunization rate (%)	Pertussis notifications	Comment
1952	0	> 100 000	Year before vaccine introduction. Death rate: 1 in 1000 cases notified
1973	80	2400	Year before 'pertussis scare'
1975	30	>100 000	After 'pertussis scare'
1978		> 65 000	12 deaths from whooping cough
1986	65	36 500	After misinterpretation of UK National Encephalopathy Study results
1988		5117	Above clarified
1989		11 646	Still 2-year peaks and troughs present
1990		16 900	7 deaths (all infants under 4 months of age)
1991	88	5207	First year of immunization targets in the GP contract. No deaths
1992	91	2309	1 death

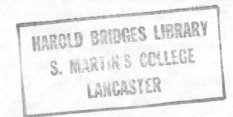

Notes

Poliomyelitis

Oral poliomyelitis vaccine (OPV)

Contraindications to vaccination

- Acute febrile illness.
- Diarrhoea and vomiting.
- Severe reaction to a previously administered dose of OPV.
- Severe hypersensitivity to penicillin, neomycin or streptomycin; in addition, to polymyxin for the Wellcome/Evans OPV.
- Immunodeficiency due to disease or treatment, and malignancy.
- Human immunodeficiency virus (HIV) positive symptomatic individuals.
- Household contacts of patients who are immunocompromised for any reason.
- Within 3 weeks of administration of a live viral vaccine — they can be given simultaneously.
- Within 3 weeks of administration of the live bacterial BCG, but may be given simultaneously. When BCG is given to infants, the primary polio immunization schedule starting at 2 months of age should not be delayed.
- Within 2 weeks from administration of the oral typhoid vaccine — until there is data about possible interaction in the gut replication.
- At 3 weeks before and 3 months after an injection of human normal immunoglobulin (HNIG). In the case of travel (as in the case of hepatitis A immunoglobulin) this contraindication may be ignored and OPV given. Where the vaccine is given as a booster, the possible inhibiting effect of immunoglobulin is less important.
- Pregnancy, although if there is a significant risk of exposure to poliomyelitis, as in the case of travel to an endemic area, the importance of vaccination may outweigh the theoretical risk to the fetus. If it is at all possible, postpone vaccination until after the 16th week of pregnancy.
- Within 3 weeks from a proposed tonsillectomy, because of the remote risk of vaccine-induced bulbar polio.

Possible side and adverse effects
OPV has been associated with paralysis in vaccine recipients and their contacts. The risk is very small and can be expressed numerically as follows:
- among first dose recipients — one case in 1 200 000;
- among contacts of first dose recipients — one case in 1000 000.

The risk after subsequent doses is greatly reduced. It is important to ensure that contacts of children receiving OPV are fully immunized.

A recent British review of all cases of paralytic poliomyelitis in England and Wales between 1985 and 1991 (*BMJ* 1992; 305: 79–82) estimated the risk of vaccine-associated paralysis to be 1.46 per million for the first dose, 0.49 for the second, 0 for the third and fourth doses, and 0.33 for the fifth.

The vaccine
OPV is a trivalent vaccine, containing live attenuated strains of poliomyelitis viruses types I, II and III, grown in cultures of human diploid cells (Wellcome/Evans) or on monkey kidney cells (SmithKline Beecham). OPV is excreted by healthy vaccinees and may persist in the faeces for up to 6 weeks — this is a possible risk for infection in immunocompromised household members.

Administration
A dose is the entire content of a monodose tube or three drops of vaccine from the 10-dose tube. It has a bitter taste, and therefore in some schools it is given on a sugar lump.

In the UK, OPV is given in infancy at the same time as routine immunization against diphtheria, tetanus and pertussis (Table 10).
- If a child vomits soon after receiving the vaccine, that dose should be repeated.
- Seroconversion: 95% of recipients.

Table 10 Childhood immunization with OPV in the UK

Primary immunization	First booster	Second booster	Further boosters
Age 2, 3, 4 months (three doses at monthly intervals)	At school entry (age 4–5)	At school leaving (age 15–19)	A: not recommended B: for those at risk, every 10+ years

Table 11 Adult immunization with OPV in the UK

Primary immunization	Boosters
Three doses at monthly intervals	A: not recommended B: for those at risk, every 10+ years including travellers to areas where polio is endemic or epidemic and health-care workers likely to be exposed to polio

- Duration of immunity: after full immunization in most people immunity is lifelong.
- In the primary course, all three doses should be given in order to ensure that each type of vaccine poliovirus is given an opportunity of establishing immunity.
- If the primary course is interrupted, it should be resumed but not repeated.
- Carers of recently immunized babies should be advised of the need of strict personal hygiene (washing hands after nappy changes) and safe disposal of soiled nappies. There is no reason to exclude a recently immunized baby from swimming pools.
- Non-immunized parents and household contacts of children receiving primary OPV immunization should be immunized against poliomyelitis at the same time as their children. If they have been fully immunized in the past, there is no need to give a booster.
- Breast feeding does not interfere with the response of the vaccine.
- The DoH advises that HIV positive asymptomatic individuals may receive OPV. It is important to note that such individuals continue to excrete the vaccine virus in their faeces for longer than normal individuals and this will apply to adults as well as infants (wash hands after nappy changes, dispose soiled nappies safely).
- A person who has been immunized with OPV may receive the injectable inactivated poliomyelitis vaccine (IPV) as a booster.
- Individuals born before 1962 (UK introduction of OPV) especially before 1956 (UK introduction of IPV) may not have been immunized and no opportunity should be missed to immunize them.
- Particular care should be taken to provide immunization to travellers abroad, to areas where poliomyelitis is endemic (developing countries).

Vaccine availability
● Wellcome/Evans Poliomyelitis Vaccine, Evans Medical Ltd, available in monodose dropper tubes. Storage: between 0 and +4°C. At room temperature (< 25°C), it can be expected to retain its potency for 1 week.
● Poliomyelitis Vaccine, SmithKline Beecham Pharmaceuticals, available in 10-dose dropper tubes. Discard any remaining vaccine at the end of a vaccinating session. Storage: between +2 and +6°C. At room temperature (< 25°C), it can be expected to retain its potency for 2 weeks. All vaccines for childhood immunization are distributed free of charge to GPs by Farillon Ltd, on behalf of the DoH.

Inactivated poliomyelitis vaccine

Contraindications to vaccination
● Acute febrile illness.
● Anaphylactic reaction to a previously administered dose of the vaccine.
● Severe hypersensitivity to neomycin.
● Pregnancy, unless there is a risk to the mother.

Possible side and adverse effects
No serious adverse effects to IPV have been documented.

The vaccine
IPV is a trivalent vaccine, containing strains of poliomyelitis viruses types I, II and III which have been inactivated with formalin. The enhanced potency poliomyelitis vaccine (eIPV) is produced in human diploid cell cultures and is highly immunogenic.

Administration
● Boosting with IPV leads to very much higher levels of polio antibodies than boosting with OPV, irrespective of whether the patient has previously been immunized with OPV or IPV.
● *Indications:*
   (a) for anybody who has refused OPV immunization but will accept IPV;
   (b) for anybody for whom the OPV is contraindicated and in particular for: (i) persons with compromised immunity who are unimmunized or partially immunized; (ii) siblings and other house-

Table 12 Administration specifications for IPV

Dose (ml)	Route	Primary immunization	Boosters
0.5	Deep SC injection	Three doses at monthly intervals	Every 5 or more years for those at risk

hold contacts of immunosuppressed individuals; (iii) HIV positive symptomatic individuals; or (iv) health-care personnel in close contact with immunosuppressed patients.

(c) in the USA the eIPV is recommended for adults because the risk of OPV-associated paralysis is slightly higher in adults than it is in children.

• There is now evidence that the incidence of OPV-associated poliovirus faecal excretion rates in children can be reduced by administering IPV for their first dose in the childhood primary immunization schedule, and then using OPV for their subsequent doses.

• In countries where the wild poliovirus is under control, such as the UK and USA, current debate concerns whether IPV should be adopted in place of OPV. This could avoid the small number of vaccine-associated paralysis cases. On the other hand, American researchers who compared different combinations of IPV and OPV in 511 infants found that strategies with OPV gave better immunity than IPV in the first 6 months of life. The current recommendation is the continuing use of OPV. When eIPV is licensed for use in combination with DTP or DT vaccine, this recommendation could change.

Vaccine availability

eIPV, produced by Connaught, available in 0.5 ml ampoules. Distributed for the DoH by Farillon Ltd. An unlicensed eIPV is available from Merieux UK Ltd on a 'named patient' basis. It is available in 0.5 ml prefilled syringes.

Storage: Between +2 and +8°C. *Do not freeze.*

Poliomyelitis infection

Infection is caused by polioviruses which are enteroviruses of which there are three types (I, II and III). Humans are the only reservoir of the virus. It is spread by contact with infected faeces or pharyngeal secretions, contaminated food and water.

The incubation period is 4–21 days. The patient is most infectious shortly before and after onset of clinical illness when the virus has colonized the throat and is excreted in large amounts in the faeces. Over 85% of children will be asymptomatic. About 10% of children will develop pyrexia without paralysis and 5% will go on to suffer headaches, vomiting, photophobia, neck stiffness and paralysis. Poliomyeloencephalitis can follow. Other children develop paralysis of the lower motor neurones (paralytic poliomyelitis).

Poliomyelitis is still prevalent in many developing countries where it occurs in epidemics. In 1988, WHO declared its intention to eradicate poliomyelitis by the year 2000. In 1974, less than 5% of children in developing countries were receiving polio immunization. By August 1991, 85% of children worldwide were receiving three doses of polio vaccine.

WHO has declared the UK as one of the countries where the indigenous poliomyelitis due to wild virus has been eliminated. In England and Wales in 1955, before the introduction of the first polio vaccine in the UK, 4000 cases of poliomyelitis were notified. Between 1985 and 1991, there were only 21 cases reported of which five were contracted abroad and 13 were vaccine-associated.

By the beginning of 1993 the vaccine uptake in children had reached 93%. Coverage in adults is not as high, therefore no opportunity in general practice should be missed to immunize all adults. Vaccine-associated contact cases could be eliminated if GPs could ensure polio immunization of all children and adults.

Table 13 Paralytic poliomyelitis rates for England and Wales

	1970–1984	1985–1991
Unknown source	30	3
Contracted abroad	11	5
Vaccine-associated:		
recipients	17	9
contacts	12	4

Haemophilus influenzae b

Contraindications to vaccination
- Acute febrile illness.
- Hypersensitivity to tetanus protein (Act-HIB) or diphtheria toxoid (HibTITER).
- Severe local (redness and swelling involving most of the circumference of the limb, at the site of the injection) or general reaction to a previously administered *Haemophilus influenzae* b (Hib) vaccine.
- Pregnancy — no data available.

Possible side and adverse effects

Local reactions
Swelling, redness and pain soon after vaccination and lasting up to 24 h in 10% of vaccinees, mainly after the first dose.

General reactions
Malaise, headaches, fever, irritability, inconsolable and high-pitched crying. Very rarely seizures. The vaccine can be generally considered as very safe.

The vaccine
The polysaccharide capsule of *Haemophilus influenzae* type b (poly-ribosylribitol phosphate, PRP) forms the basis of the Hib vaccine. Unfortunately, PRP alone provokes a poor antibody response in younger children (under 18 months of age) who are at most risk. Linking the capsular polysaccharide to a protein such as diphtheria or tetanus toxoid, improves considerably the immunogenic response, especially in children less than 1 year of age. It provokes higher titres of antibody (predominantly IgG) and a longer lasting immune response because of stimulation of memory cells. There are three *H. influenzae* type b conjugate vaccines licensed in the UK of which Pedvax (at the time of going to press, summer 1994) was not as yet available.

Table 14 *Haemophilus influenzae* b vaccines

Trade name	Abbreviation	Carrier protein	Manufacturer	Availability (1994)
Act-HIB	PRP-T	Tetanus toxoid	Merieux	Yes
HibTITER	HbOC	Mutant diphtheria toxin	Lederle	Yes
Pedvax	PRP-OMP	Outer membrane protein complex of *Neisseria meningitidis*	Merck Sharp & Dohme	No

Administration

● The primary course consists of three doses of the vaccine with a 4-week interval between each dose. It is administered only to babies under the age of 13 months and Act-HIB is the vaccine of choice (which may also be used for the 'catch-up' programme). This vaccine can also be given by deep SC injection.

● Children immunized for the first time aged 1–4 years receive only one dose and HibTITER is recommended (may also be used for the primary course). This has been necessary as the vaccine was only introduced into the British first year schedule of immunization in October 1992.

● Over the age of 4 years, routine immunization is not recommended by the DoH.

● The vaccines are not interchangeable because of the different carrier proteins they use. If children under the age of 1 year are started on a course with one vaccine, and the course is interrupted, it should be resumed irrespective of the interval and with the same vaccine. If that brand of vaccine is not available, the whole course should be repeated with a different brand of vaccine.

● The Hib vaccine can be given at the same time as the MMR, or polio and triple vaccination (DTP), but should be given in the opposite thigh (the site at which each vaccine has been given should be recorded).

Table 15 Administration specifications for Hib vaccine

Age at first immunization (months)	Dose (ml)	Route	No. of doses	Interval	Booster
2–12	0.5	IM	3	4 weeks	None
13–48	0.5	IM	1	—	None

Practices usually agree that DTP is given in the left thigh, while Hib vaccine is given in the right.

● Revaccination of children over the age of 1 year and adults with the conjugate vaccine is not currently recommended in the UK.

● Vaccination of babies at 2, 3 and 4 months has been included in the GP target payments as from July 1994.

● Vaccine efficacy is estimated at 98% for infants immunized from 2 months of age. Antibody titres greater than $1\mu g/ml$ are thought to correlate with long-term protection.

● The Hib vaccine is only effective against encapsulated strains of *H. influenzae* type b, therefore it will not protect against conditions such as otitis media and acute exacerbations of chronic bronchitis caused by non-capsulated strains.

● The vaccine seems to protect both inoculated and non-inoculated children, possibly through a reduction in asymptomatic carriage rates.

● The tetanus and diphtheria proteins in the vaccine do not replace the need for routine tetanus and diphtheria immunization.

● Premature babies should be given Hib vaccine at 2, 3 and 4 months of age without adjusting for prematurity.

● The DoH advises the following action in the case of contact with a patient with invasive Hib disease:

(a) in a nursery, playgroup or crèche, all unimmunized children under 4 years of age should be immunized;

(b) unimmunized household contacts under 4 years of age should be immunized. Rifampicin prophylaxis should be given to all household contacts (except pregnant women). Rifampicin dosage is 20 mg/kg once daily (with a maximum daily dose of 600 mg) for 4 days;

(c) the index case should also be immunized, irrespective of age; and

(d) post-splenectomy, and especially before if it is an elective procedure.

● In the USA indications for the conjugate Hib vaccine are widened to include children over 4 years of age who are at high risk of Hib disease, not only those who have had a splenectomy, but also children treated for malignancy and those with sickle cell disease and HIV.

Vaccine availability

● Act-HIB, Merieux UK Ltd, available as single vial of lyophilized vaccine plus one syringe of diluent (0.5 ml).

● HibTITER, Lederle Laboratories, available as monodose vial, containing 0.72 ml to allow easy withdrawal of the 0.5 ml dose.

All vaccines for childhood immunization are distributed free of charge to GPs by Farillon Ltd, on behalf of the DoH.

Storage. Between +2 and +8°C. *Do not freeze.*

Haemophilus influenzae type b infection

Haemophilus influenzae is a Gram-negative coccobacillus, with six antigenically distinct capsular types (a–f) as well as non-encapsulated strains. It was discovered by Pfeiffer in 1892.

The non-encapsulated strains cause infections that are non-preventable, such as otitis media and bronchitis. They can be found as asymptomatic in the throat of over 60% of children.

Type b accounts for more than 95% of the encapsulated *H. influenzae* disease. It causes meningitis (60% of cases), epiglottitis (15%), septicaemia, septic arthritis, pneumonia, empyema, pericarditis, osteomyelitis and cellulitis. About 2–8% of meningitis cases end in death, and 10–30% in long-term neurological sequelae such as seizures, intellectual impairment, vision or hearing loss, motor dysfunction and behavioural alterations.

More than 85% of Hib disease cases occur in children under the age of 5 years with peak incidence of Hib meningitis occurring in children between 6 and 12 months and epiglottitis in children aged 2–4 years old.

The source of infection is the upper respiratory tract where type b organisms can be recovered from 1–5% of children. The incubation period is unknown. It affects 1 in 600 children aged under 5 with a case fatality rate of 5%.

In England and Wales, there were 869 laboratory reports of Hib disease in 1983, rising steadily to 1259 reports in 1989 — the Hib vaccine was introduced in the UK in 1992. During that year there were 484 laboratory reports of Hib infection in England and Wales (341 in babies under 1 year old) while in 1993 the number of reports dropped to 168 (65 in babies under 1 year old). An average of 90% of children under 12 months received three doses of the vaccine in 1993.

Countries where Hib vaccine has been introduced into routine immunization schedules such as Finland, have seen a dramatic reduction in cases of Hib disease and the sequelae from it. It seems that this success is being repeated in the UK.

Measles/mumps/rubella combined

Contraindications to vaccination
● Acute febrile illness.
● Within 3 weeks of administration of another live virus vaccine or the live bacterial BCG vaccine.
● Within 3 months of administration of blood or plasma transfusion or HNIG (if the vaccine is given, check seroconversion 8 weeks later).
● Malignancy and immunodeficiency by disease or therapy. It should not be given to an immunodeficient child (for definition see p. 10). HIV disease is not a contraindication.
● Untreated tuberculosis — patients with active tuberculosis should at least be on treatment if vaccination is administered. If there is a need for tuberculin skin testing, it should be performed on the day of MMR vaccination or 4–6 weeks later — measles vaccination can temporarily suppress tuberculin reactivity and render the test temporarily negative.
● Pregnancy and at least 1 month before (the manufacturer advises 3 months before, the DoH 1 month before).
● Severe reaction to a previously administered dose of the vaccine.
● Severe hypersensitivity to neomycin.
● Anaphylactic hypersensitivity to hen's eggs.
● Children below 12 months of age should not normally be vaccinated as persisting passively acquired maternal antibodies can interfere with their ability to respond to the vaccine and they may not develop sustained antibody levels when later reimmunized. If it is necessary to give the vaccine to a child under the age of 12 months, a second dose should be given at 15 months and ideally seroconversion should be checked.
● If a child with a cold is vaccinated, seroconversion should be checked as there is evidence of a failure rate of up to 21% to respond to the measles vaccine in such cases.

Possible side and adverse reactions

Local reactions
Swelling, redness and pain at the injection site.

General reactions
These are similar to those expected from administration of monovalent vaccines given separately. The attenuated vaccine viruses are not thought to be transmissible to contacts when a rash or other side effects occur in a vaccinee.

Reactions to the measles component of the vaccine
- Transient rash in 5% of vaccinees.
- Fever over 39.4°C in 5–15% of vaccinees, between 5 and 12 days after vaccination, lasting 1–2 days (on occasions up to 5 days).
- Malaise, coryza, pharyngitis, headaches, nausea, vomiting and diarrhoea with or without a rash.
- Febrile convulsions, usually at 6–14 days, in 1 in 1000–9000 doses of the vaccine. It may be higher in children with previous convulsions or a family history of epilepsy or febrile convulsions. No long-term sequelae of post-vaccination febrile convulsions have been reported (incidence of febrile convulsions in natural measles is about 1 in 200). Such children should be immunized and the parents should be warned about the timing and the risks, and advised on ways to control fever, including the use of paracetamol in the period of 5 to at least 10 days after immunization. Parents of very susceptible children may have to be supplied with, and instructed in the use of, rectal diazepam to administer while awaiting the GP to arrive in cases where post-vaccination convulsions occur.
- Encephalitis and encephalopathy occurring within 30 days after vaccination have been reported in about 1 in 1000 000 doses of measles vaccine (incidence after natural measles is 1 in 1000–5000 cases).
- Subacute sclerosing panencephalitis (SSPE) is estimated to occur in 1 in 1000 000 doses. Some of these children may have had unrecognized measles disease before vaccination. SSPE can affect children who have had measles infection in the past (6–22 in 1 000 000 cases) and in the great majority the onset is in the first two decades of life — insidious onset, intellectual deterioration, rigidity, spasticity and death within a year or two. It can be concluded that measles vaccine protects children from SSPE by preventing measles infection.

Reaction to the mumps component of the vaccine
- Transient rash, pruritus and purpura are uncommon and of brief duration.
- Parotitis in about 1% of vaccinees, 3 or more weeks after vaccination.

- Orchitis may rarely occur and retrobulbar neuritis very rarely.
- Meningoencephalitis occurring 14–30 days after immunization is mild, and the sequelae are rare. At present only the Jeryl Lynn mumps strain-containing MMR vaccine is licensed in the UK. Such a complication is expected extremely rarely and put at 1 in 1 800 000 doses. The DoH withdrew all MMR vaccines containing the Urabe Am 9 strain in September 1992, as the rate of meningoencephalitis was reported in 1 in 300 000 doses of these vaccines (this complication after natural mumps infection is reported to occur at a rate of 1 in 400 cases).

Reactions to the rubella component of the vaccine
- Rash, fever and lymphadenopathy at 5–12 days in a small percentage of children.
- Thrombocytopenia is seen occasionally and is usually self-limiting.
- Transient peripheral neuritis, paraesthesiae and pain in the upper and lower limbs can rarely occur 3 days to 3 months after immunization.
- Mild episodes of joint and limb symptoms can occur especially in girls and children under the age of 5 years.
- Arthritis and arthralgia occur in up to 3% of children and up to 20% of adults receiving the vaccine. They are more marked and of longer duration in adults. Joint involvement begins 7–21 days after vaccination and is generally transient. Adults seldom have to limit their work activities. Symptoms may persist for months or, on rare occasions, for years but the aetiological relationship to vaccination is unclear.
- Polyneuropathy, including Guillain–Barré syndrome have been reported rarely and in isolated cases.

The vaccine
It contains Enders' attenuated Edmonston strain measles, Jeryl Lynn strain mumps and Wistar RA 27/3 strain of live attenuated rubella virus.

Administration
- The vaccine should be reconstituted only with the diluent supplied and should be used within 1 h after reconstitution.
- The injection site is the upper arm, though infants receive it at the anterolateral thigh.
- Seroconversion occurs in 95% for measles, 96% for mumps and 99% for rubella. Incorrectly stored vaccine and exposure of the vaccine to light (which can inactivate the measles component) may cause failure of the vaccine to protect.

Table 16 Administration specifications for MMR vaccine

Age	Dose (ml)	Route	Reimmunization	Boosters
Children over 12 months and adults	0.5	SC/IM	Only if given before 12 months of age	None recommended in the UK

- Duration of immunity: administration of the MMR vaccine under the age of 12 months is avoided in the UK because of possible interference in the uptake of the measles vaccine by persisting passively acquired maternal antibodies against measles. However, up to 30% of African children get measles before 9 months of age, therefore, WHO recommends that in countries with a high incidence of measles in infancy, measles vaccine should be given at 6 months of age.

- Up to 5% of immunized and the small number of unvaccinated young children remain susceptible to measles disease. Measles susceptibility for 11–14 year olds in the UK is increasing. In the USA where there is a much longer history of MMR vaccination, outbreaks of measles have occurred in immunized populations. However, most cases can be attributed to primary immunization at or before 12 months, or the expected 2–5% rate of failed seroconversion with primary immunization, rather than waning immunity, although a small percentage of vaccinated individuals may lose protection after several years. An increasing number of cases of measles in the USA are attributable to exposure in foreign countries. The USA, therefore, recommend a second dose (booster) of MMR at entrance to middle school or junior high school, usually at the age of 11 or 12. Other countries with a similar policy to the USA include Sweden, Finland, Poland, Australia and New Zealand. Such a policy also provides additional immunization for rubella and mumps.

- Vaccine-induced antibodies to rubella are detectable 18 + years after immunization in the UK. As girls in Britain are now vaccinated at 15 months, there may be a case for a booster at high school entry age. This suggestion takes into consideration the true rubella vaccine failure rate estimated at less than 2% with its potential consequences (congenital rubella).

- In order to reduce the effect of vaccine failures and boost immunity, there is a need in the UK to also introduce a booster dose of MMR. This, as yet, is not recommended by the DoH.

- The single-dose MMR at 15 months may be shifting the occurrence of mumps to older age groups.
- MMR should be given irrespective of history of previous measles, mumps or rubella infection. Vaccination is not harmful for individuals already immune.
- The MMR vaccine is protective if given within 72 h of contact with measles. The same is not observed for mumps and rubella as the antibody response to them is too slow for effective prophylaxis after exposure.
- *Indications:* in the UK, the MMR vaccine is recommended for:

    (a) children aged 12–15 months;

    (b) children of any age not previously immunized and especially children with chronic conditions such as cystic fibrosis, congenital heart or kidney disease, Down's syndrome, failure to thrive or in residential or day care;

    (c) non-immune adults that request it, especially those in long-term institutional care;

    (d) HIV infected children.

- MMR vaccine uptake among 2 year olds in England and Wales reached 92% in November 1992.
- Children and adults with contraindications to the MMR vaccine such as with malignancies or the immunosuppressed by disease or treatment, or children under 12 months, should receive HNIG IM (Table 17) as soon as possible and not later than 6 days after exposure to measles. If MMR is not further contraindicated, 3 months should be allowed to pass before vaccination is undertaken.
- HNIG should also be given to pregnant women with confirmed rubella infection, for whom therapeutic abortion is unacceptable. It must be given as soon as possible after exposure, at the dose of 750 mg IM.

Table 17 Dosage of HNIG in measles

Age	Dose (mg)
To modify an attack	
under 1 year	100
1 year and over	250
To prevent an attack	
under 1 year	250
1–2 years	500
3 years and over	750

- HNIG can be obtained from the Central Public Health Laboratory Services, Bio Products Laboratory, Immuno Ltd (Gammabulin), Kabi Pharmacia (Kabiglobulin), The Laboratories, Belfast City Hospital and the Blood Transfusion Services, Scotland (see p. 215).
- HNIG is supplied as 250 and 750 mg single-dose vials.

Storage: Between 0 and +4°C.

Vaccine availability

MMR II, Merck Sharp & Dohme Ltd are product licence holders. The vaccine is distributed to GPs on behalf of the DoH, free of charge, directly by Farillon Ltd. Available as single-dose vials of freeze-dried vaccine powder with diluent.

Storage: Between +2 and +8°C. *Do not freeze diluent.* Protect from light.

Measles

Contraindications to vaccination
Same as for MMR vaccine (see p. 49) with the addition of a history of severe hypersensitivity to polymyxin.

Possible side and adverse effects
Same as for MMR vaccine (see p. 50).

The vaccine
Monovalent freeze-dried preparation of live attenuated virus of the Schwarz strain, prepared on chick embryo cell cultures.

Administration
The vaccine requires reconstitution with water for injection provided by the manufacturer. Once reconstituted, it should be allowed to stand for about a minute and then the suspension should be mixed by withdrawing into the syringe and expelling back into the vial. Alcohol should not be used, but if it is necessary for the skin to be cleaned prior to injection the alcohol should be allowed to evaporate dry before the vaccine is given.

Adults and children over 12 months should be given 0.5 ml of the reconstituted vaccine, by deep SC or IM injection. If given to a child under 12 months, a second dose (MMR) should be given at 15 months (see p. 49).

Indications
- Susceptible, unimmunized adults or children exposed to measles should receive the vaccine within 72 h of exposure. An acceptable alternative for individuals in whom measles vaccine is contraindicated, is to use HNIG (see p. 53). HNIG can prevent or modify measles infection if given within 6 days of exposure. HNIG should not be given with measles vaccine.
- Unimmunized, susceptible adults or children with chronic conditions such as cystic fibrosis, congenital heart or kidney disease, failure to thrive, Down's syndrome, and those patients in residential or day care.

- Susceptible travellers abroad.
- Children whose parents refuse to allow vaccination with the rubella and/or mumps components of MMR vaccine but will allow vaccination against measles.
- In the case of a measles epidemic where there is a decision to vaccinate children under 12 months. Such children should receive the MMR vaccine at the age of 15 or more months.
- MMR (therefore measles) vaccine is currently recommended for HIV infected children.

Vaccine availability
Mevilin-L, Evans Medical Ltd, currently available from the manufacturers on a 'named patient' basis as a 10-dose vial with a 5 ml ampoule of water for injections.

Storage: Between +2 and +8°C. *Do not freeze diluent.* Protect from light.

Measles infection
Measles is an acute highly transmissible viral infection, has a worldwide distribution and humans are the only reservoir. It is a single-stranded RNA virus with one antigenic type, classified as a morbillivirus. It is transmitted by direct contact with infectious droplets. The incubation period is 8–12 days from exposure to onset of symptoms and 14 days to appearance of the rash. Patients are contagious for 1–2 days before the onset of symptoms and 3–5 days before the rash.

Clinical features include the pathognomonic Koplik spots, conjunctivitis, coryza, pharyngitis, fever and rash. Complications include otitis media (5%), chest infection (3–7%), febrile convulsions (1 in 200), encephalitis (1 in 1000–5000) and SSPE (6–22 in 1 000 000 cases). Complications are reported in the UK in 5–10% of cases (Table 18). The fatality rate from measles is 1 in 6000 cases.

Measles infection during pregnancy increases the risk of miscarriage, premature labour and low birthweight. Pregnant women are 6.4 times as likely to die of measles complications than non-pregnant women with measles. HNIG should be considered for unvaccinated/susceptible pregnant women in contact with measles (see p. 53).

Notification of measles began in England and Wales in 1940 and measles vaccine was introduced in 1968. This was associated with a dramatic reduction of notifications to the Office of Population Censuses and Surveys (OPCS) of cases and deaths from measles. Further improvement was seen when in 1988 the MMR vaccine was introduced.

Table 18 Comparison of complications

	Measles infection	Measles vaccine
Pyrexia and rash	Almost 100%	5–10%
Febrile convulsions	1 in 200	1 in 1000–9000
Encephalitis	1 in 1000–5000	1 in 1000000
	15% fatal;	
	20–40% residual	
	neurological sequelae	
SSPE	6–22 in 1000000	< 1 in 1000000

Table 19 Measles infection (England and Wales)

Year	Notifications/annum	Deaths/annum
1940–1968	160000–800000	1000 (1940)
		90 (1968)
Mid-1970s	50000–180000	
1985	97400	10
1988	86001	
1989	26222	
1990	13302	1
1991	9201	1*
1992	10268	2*
1993	9612	

* Unconfirmed at time of going to press.

Notes

Mumps

Contraindications to vaccination
Same as for MMR vaccine (see p. 49).

Possible side and adverse effects
Same as for MMR vaccine (see p. 50).

The vaccine
Monovalent live attenuated virus vaccine, prepared in chick embryo cell culture from the Jeryl Lynn strain (so named after the patient from whom the virus was initially recovered).

The vaccine should be reconstituted with the diluent provided. Shake gently to mix and withdraw the entire vial content into a syringe. Use within 1 h of reconstitution. Protect from light.

Administration
- Adults and children over 12 months: the total volume of reconstituted vaccine (0.5 ml) injected SC, preferably into the outer aspect of the upper arm.
- It is not recommended for children under 12 months of age as persisting passively acquired maternal mumps antibodies can interfere with the immune response to the vaccine.
- Seroconversion occurs in approximately 97% of susceptible children and 93% of susceptible adults.
- Duration of immunity is long-lasting and probably lifelong. There is no need to give boosters. Revaccination is only recommended if there is evidence that initial immunization was ineffective. If given to a person who already has naturally acquired or vaccine-induce immunity, it is not associated with adverse effects.
- The vaccine will not protect when given after exposure to mumps infection.
- HNIG is no longer recommended for post-exposure protection (there is no evidence that it is effective). Mumps-specific HNIG is no longer available in the UK.

Indications:

● For unvaccinated children over 12 months of age whose parents refuse to allow immunization against measles and/or rubella but will allow vaccination against mumps to be given.

● Susceptible children and adults (lack of documented mumps vaccination or infection, lack of serological evidence of immunity) particularly those approaching puberty.

● Susceptible travellers abroad.

● M M R (therefore mumps) vaccine is currently recommended for H I V infected children.

Vaccine availability

Mumpsvax, Merck Sharp & Dohme, available as a single-dose vial of lyophilized vaccine with an ampoule containing diluent.

Storage: Between + 2 and + 8°C. *Do not freeze diluent.* Protect from light.

Mumps infection

Mumps is a generalized infection, caused by the mumps virus which is a myxovirus. 'To mump' is an old word meaning to look glum and weary, which patients with parotid swelling do.

Humans are the only reservoir of the virus which is transmitted by direct contact with infectious droplets. The incubation period is 14–21 days and mumps is transmissible from 7 days prior to the onset of parotid swelling to 9 days after onset.

Approximately one-third of infections do not cause parotid gland enlargement. Parotitis is usually accompanied by fever. The most serious aspect of mumps is the complications:

● Epididymo-orchitis in as many as 38% of post-pubertal boys and men with clinical illness, but sterility rarely occurs.

● Meningoencephalitis in 1 in 400 cases.

● Pancreatitis

● Myocarditis.

● Arthritis.

● Thyroiditis.

● Mastitis.

● Oophoritis.

● Renal involvement.

● Hearing impairment.

During the first trimester of pregnancy it can increase the rate of miscarriage up to 27%. Epidemics of mumps have occurred at 3-yearly intervals in England and Wales.

Before the introduction of MMR vaccine, mumps was the commonest cause of viral meningitis in children, a common cause of permanent unilateral deafness at any age, and was responsible for about 1200 hospital admissions each year in England and Wales.

Mumps was made a notifiable disease in the UK in October 1988 to coincide with the introduction of the MMR vaccine. There was a marked impact on the incidence of mumps notified to the OPCS following the introduction of the MMR vaccine, with a 79.4% drop in notifications during 1990 compared with 1989 figures. The 3-yearly epidemic cycle was also interrupted (Tables 20 and 21).

Table 20 Notification of mumps infection in the UK

Year	
1989	20713
1990	4277
1991	2794
1992	2171
1993	2073

Table 21 Deaths due to mumps infection in the UK

Year	Deaths/annum
1962–1981	4.7
1982–1988	2.9
1989	1
1990–1992	0

Notes

Rubella

Contraindications to vaccination

Same as for M M R vaccine (see p. 49) with the addition of a history of severe hypersensitivity to polymyxin for the Evans rubella vaccine, and the exception of anaphylactic hypersensitivity to hen's eggs — the vaccine is not prepared on chick embryo cell cultures.

Possible side and adverse effects

Same as for M M R vaccine (see p. 51).

The vaccine

All rubella vaccines available in the U K contain the Wistar R A 27/3 strain grown in human diploid cells, and come with diluent.

Administration

Once reconstituted using the diluent provided, the vaccine should be used within 1 h. The dose for all ages is 0.5 ml given by S C or I M injection.

• Seroconversion occurs in 95–98% of vaccinees. True vaccine failure rate is estimated at less than 2% if the vaccine is administered correctly.

• Vaccine-induced antibodies to rubella are detectable 18 + years after immunization in the U K. Immunity for those who seroconvert is probably lifelong. On the other hand the potential consequences of rubella vaccine failure are substantial (i.e. congenital rubella), therefore an additional dose of rubella vaccine should provide an added safeguard against such failures. This second dose could be in the form of a booster dose of the M M R vaccine at secondary school entry, taking into consideration that the first M M R vaccine is given at the age of 15 months. As of yet, the DoH has not recommended this schedule.

• The administration of rubella vaccine to a person with either vaccine-induced or naturally acquired immunity is not associated with an increased risk of adverse reactions. It is not always necessary to serotest non-pregnant women before vaccination, especially if this means a better acceptance of the rubella vaccine.

• It is not recommended for children under 12 months of age, as persisting passively acquired maternal rubella antibodies can interfere with the immune response to the vaccine.

- The vaccine will not protect when given after exposure to rubella infection.
- HNIG should be given to pregnant women with confirmed rubella infection, for whom therapeutic abortion is unacceptable. It must be given as soon as possible after exposure, at a dose of 750 mg IM. Such action could reduce the likelihood of clinical symptoms and possibly reduce the risk to the fetus. (For HNIG availability see p. 53.)
- Screening for rubella immunity: in the USA the recommendation is that patients who do not have a documented history of vaccination, should be given the choice of serological test or vaccination. In the UK the DoH recommends a different approach whereby all women of childbearing age should be screened (serotested) for rubella antibody and immunized where necessary. Screening can be done at every opportunity such as at family planning, ante-natal care, infertility clinics, and so on. Further, it is recommended that women are screened at every pregnancy, and on request when pregnancy is contemplated, irrespective of a previous positive rubella antibody result. It is important to note that apart from possible laboratory errors where a negative result is reported as positive, 25% of the small number of women currently being infected during pregnancy had been reported to be rubella immune in the past.
- Anti-D immunoglobulin if required by a rhesus negative post-natal patient, who also requires rubella vaccine, could be given at the same time though using a different site and a separate syringe (although it has been established that it does not interfere with the antibody response to the vaccine). On the other hand, blood or plasma transfusion could inhibit antibody response, therefore it is necessary to check antibody response 8 weeks after vaccination and transfusion.
- Although some vaccinees shed small amounts of vaccine virus from the pharynx, such virus is not transmissible, therefore there is no need to defer immunization of the contacts of pregnant women.
- Nursing mothers immunized with live attenuated RA 27/3 strain rubella vaccine may transmit the virus via breast milk. In those babies with serological evidence of rubella, none showed clinical disease.
- Rubella vaccination should be avoided during pregnancy and 1 month before pregnancy. The current advice is that the risk of rubella-associated damage following inadvertent rubella vaccination in pregnancy or shortly before is low, therefore termination of pregnancy

should not be routinely recommended in these circumstances. The maximum theoretical risk of fetal damage following rubella vaccination in the critical period (1 week before and 1 month after conception) is estimated at 4.4%. In the cases of inadvertent rubella vaccination during pregnancy that continued to delivery, notified between 1981 and 1992, no child was born with defects attributable to congenital infection, although in four out of 14 infants rubella-specific IgM antibody was detected (similar findings in the USA). 1990 saw the lowest rate of termination because of rubella immunization in pregnancy — just five cases (738 in 1972).

● Rubella reinfection can occur in women with both natural and vaccine-induced antibody. When it occurs in pregnancy the risk to the fetus cannot be calculated precisely but it is considered to be low. The criteria for confirming a diagnosis of maternal rubella reinfection requires evidence of either two or more previous antibody positive laboratory reports, or a documented history of rubella immunization followed by at least one antibody positive report. Between 1990 and 1992 there were 37 women with confirmed rubella infection in pregnancy. Of these, nine were considered to have a confirmed or probable reinfection according to the above criteria. Eight of these women continued with their pregnancies and no evidence of fetal infection was found in the six infants tested (two were not followed up) (*Comm Dis Rep* 1993; 3 (3)).

Indications
● For all girls aged 10–14 years who have not previously received the MMR vaccine. A history of rubella should be ignored.
● Non-pregnant women of childbearing age who are seronegative. They should avoid becoming pregnant for at least 1 month after vaccination.
● Post-natal patients who have been found in the ante-natal clinics to be seronegative. Vaccination should take place in the post-natal ward or during the immediate post-natal period. The mother should be warned of the need to use adequate contraception for 1 month after vaccination.
● All health-care staff, both male and female, who work in ante-natal clinics, GP surgeries or anywhere else where they may come into contact with pregnant patients.
● Female immigrants who have entered the UK and because of their age are not likely to have been vaccinated at school in the UK.

- MMR (therefore rubella) vaccine is currently recommended for HIV infected children.
- Children whose parents refuse to allow vaccination with the measles and/or mumps component of MMR vaccine but will allow vaccination against rubella.
- A group of women whom GPs are well advised to target are Asian and Oriental women. Of the women giving birth to congenitally infected infants between 1987 and 1992, 24% were Asian or Oriental of whom at least three (out of 22) acquired the infection abroad.

Vaccine availability
- Rubella Vaccine Live BP, Evans Medical Ltd.
- Ervevax, SmithKline Beecham Pharmaceuticals.
- Rubavax, Merieux UK Ltd.
All available in single-dose vial of freeze-dried vaccine with diluent.

Storage. Between +2 and +8°C. *Do not freeze diluent.* Protect from light.

Rubella infection
Rubella is also known as German measles. The word German is probably derived from the word 'germane', meaning something akin to or very like something else. In this sense German measles means something very like ordinary measles.

Rubella is a mild disease characterized by an erythematous maculopapular discreet rash, cervical lymphadenopathy, low-grade fever and transient polyarthralgia. Thrombocytopenia and encephalitis are rare complications. Rubella infection in 25–50% of cases is asymptomatic.

Rubella has a worldwide distribution with humans as the only reservoir. It is transmitted through direct or droplet contact from nasopharyngeal secretions. The incubation period is 14–21 days and the infectivity period from 1 week before until 5–7 days after the onset of rash. The peak incidence of infection is in late winter and early spring.

The significance of rubella lies almost entirely in its ability to cause fetal malformation or death if contracted by pregnant women — congenital rubella syndrome (CRS).

The risk of fetal damage is estimated at 90% in the first 10 weeks of pregnancy. It then declines to 10– 20% by 16 weeks. In the second half of pregnancy fetal damage is rare.

Possible fetal defects are as follows:
- Cardiac — patent ductus arteriosus, atrial or ventricular septal defects, pulmonary artery stenosis.
- Auditory — sensorineural deafness.
- Ophthalmological — cataracts, glaucoma, microphthalmia, pigmentary retinopathy.
- Neurological — mental retardation, meningoencephalitis, microcephaly.
- Other findings can be purpuric like skin lesions, thrombocytopenia, jaundice, hepatomegaly, splenomegaly or growth retardation.

Infants with CRS can continue to shed virus in nasopharyngeal secretions and urine for a year or more and therefore can transmit infection.

Attempts at elimination of rubella in the UK, Europe and North America depend upon an ability to immunize almost, and if possible all, young children of both sexes and thus create conditions of herd immunity. This should stop the rubella virus circulating and thus prevent non-immune women acquiring the infection. This policy relies on sufficient numbers of children (over 90%) being immunized.

Preventing fetal infection and consequent CRS is the primary objective of rubella immunization. Rubella vaccination was introduced in the UK in 1970 primarily for schoolgirls aged 11–13 years. In October 1988, the MMR vaccine was introduced for all children, with primary immunization at 15 months. By 1992, the MMR vaccine uptake in England and Wales reached 92% among 2 year olds.

The high uptake of MMR vaccine has had a major impact on rubella susceptibility in children under 5 years old, with interruption of the epidemic cycle as well as the occurrence of fetal infection (Table 22).

Table 22 Numbers of congenitally infected infants in the UK

Year	
1987–1989	75
1990–1992	19

Rubella became a notifiable disease in the UK in October 1988 to coincide with the introduction of the MMR vaccine. There has been a dramatic reduction of rubella cases notified to the OPCS (Table 23).

Table 23 Number of notified rubella cases in the U K

Year	
1988	Not notifiable
1989	24570
1990	11491
1991	6921
1992	5434
1993	9493*

* This upsurge of notifications has not as yet been explained.

Tuberculosis — BCG

Contraindications to vaccination
- Acute febrile illness.
- Septic skin conditions or burns at the proposed vaccination site.
- Generalized eczema — may be given during remission or to an eczema-free arm.
- Malignancy.
- Immunodeficiency by disease or treatment (including systemic steroids) or deficiency (e.g. hypogammaglobulinaemia).
- HIV positive individuals, including infants born to HIV positive mothers (in countries where the risk of tuberculosis is high, WHO recommends that asymptomatic HIV infected children should receive BCG at birth or shortly after).
- Tuberculin positive reactors (apart from Heaf grade 1 reactors who can be regarded as tuberculin negative).
- Within 3 weeks (minimum 10 days) of administration of another live vaccine but may be given simultaneously and at a different site.
- Pregnancy, particularly at early stages. However, where there is a significant risk of infection, the importance of vaccination may outweigh the possible risk to the fetus. If possible, postpone vaccination until after delivery.
- Patients who are receiving prophylactic doses of antituberculous drugs.
- The ID route must not be used for the percutaneous BCG vaccine.
- No further immunization should be given in the arm used for BCG vaccination for at least 3 months because of the risk of regional lymphadenitis.

Possible side and adverse effects

Local reactions
A papule is expected at the site of the vaccination within 2–6 weeks. Over time the papule flattens and widens with some scaling and crusting. A discharging ulcer may occur at the vaccination site, usually due to

either inadvertent SC injection or excessive dose. If allowed to dry without irritation from clothes or dressings/plasters, the ulcer usually heals leaving only a small scar. Rarely, an abscess may form.

At 6 weeks after BCG vaccination there should be a scar of a diameter measuring at least 4 mm. Perform a post-BCG tuberculin test on any vaccinee who shows unsatisfactory or no reaction, and if negative, revaccinate.

Some individuals (especially of some racial groups) are more prone to keloid formation even when given at the recommended site for vaccination (the insertion of the deltoid muscle). Sites higher than those recommended or elsewhere are associated with higher risk of keloid formation.

General reactions

Adenitis (usually minor) with or without suppuration and discharge is not uncommon. Very rarely lupoid skin reaction and anaphylaxis may occur.

The risk of BCG vaccine-disseminated infection is very rare indeed, estimated at less than 1 in 1 000 000, and suppurative adenitis 100-4300 in 100 000 vaccinees. The risk of post-BCG vaccination osteitis is put at 25 in 100 000.

The vaccine

Two BCG vaccines are available and they both contain a live attenuated strain derived from *Mycobacterium bovis* (known to protect against tuberculosis). The potency of the ID BCG vaccine is 10 times less than that of percutaneous BCG vaccine.

Administration

ID BCG vaccine

This is available freeze-dried in rubber-capped vials with diluent in a separate ampoule. The vaccine suspension is prepared by adding 1 ml of diluent to the 10-dose vial (5 ml to the 50-dose vial). Only the diluent supplied with the vial should be used. Do not shake or mix. Allow to stand for 1 min, then draw into the syringe (a disposable tuberculin syringe and needle are ideal) twice to ensure homogeneity. It should then be protected from light and used within 4 h.

If alcohol is used to swab the skin and/or the rubber bung of the vial, it should be allowed to evaporate.

Table 24 Administration specifications for ID BCG vaccine

Age	Dose (ml)	Route
Adults and children over 3 months	0.1	Strictly ID
Infants under 3 months	0.05	Strictly ID

Percutaneous BCG vaccine

This is used only for neonates, infants and very young children (not recommended for older children) as an alternative to the ID route. A modified Heaf gun is used. Such a multiple punctive apparatus is equipped with not less than 20 needles giving reliable penetration of the skin to a depth of 2 mm, and is properly sterilized each time after use according to the manufacturer's instructions. Disposable heads are also available.

The same precautions about the use of alcohol on the skin and rubber bung of the vial apply as mentioned above.

0.3 ml of water for injections or sodium chloride injection BP is added to the 10-multidose vial and the suspension, without being shaken, is allowed to stand for 1 min. With a glass rod, platinum loop or spatula, a small amount (about 0.03 ml) is transferred onto the skin and immediately punctured with the multiple puncture apparatus. The vaccine suspension should be protected from light and used within 4 h.

General

● The site of injection of both vaccines is the insertion of the deltoid muscle near the middle of the upper arm.

● Post-BCG active immunity is evident (Mantoux positive) after 8–14 weeks from vaccination.

● The efficacy in British children is approximately 70–80% (80% observed in the British Medical Research Council trial).

Indications: in the UK, the DoH recommends BCG immunization (*Immunization against Infectious Disease*, HMSO, 1992) for the following provided they are tuberculin negative (except babies under 3 months of age who may be immunized without prior skin testing):

(a) schoolchildren aged 10–13 years;

(b) all students;

(c) newly born babies and children whose parents request BCG immunization;

(d) adults who request BCG immunization; and

(e) those at higher risk, e.g. (i) health-care staff who may come into contact with infectious patients or material; (ii) veterinary and other staff; (iii) contacts of cases with active tuberculosis; (iv) immigrants from countries with high prevalence of tuberculosis, their children and their infants born subsequently in the UK; and (v) those intending to stay in Asia, Africa, Central or South America for more than 1 month.

• In addition to the above groups, other at-risk groups are people living in poor and overcrowded conditions, vagrants (alcohol appears to predispose to tuberculosis) and IV drug users.

• Neonatally administered BCG is highly effective in preventing severe tuberculosis infection in children. The British Paediatric Association and DoH recommend vaccination of the following groups:

(a) babies of Asian and other immigrant families with high rates of tuberculosis;

(b) infants who reside in or travel to areas of high risk;

(c) infants with a family history of tuberculosis in the past 5 years; and

(d) infants in contact with active pulmonary tuberculosis.

Tuberculin testing and BCG

• Patients develop cell-mediated immunity 6–8 weeks after *Mycobacterium tuberculosis* infection which can be demonstrated using ID injection of purified tuberculin protein. This shows whether the patient has ever come into contact with a *Mycobacterium* species and has developed sensitivity.

• Skin tests for tuberculosis now used in the UK are the Mantoux and Heaf tests. Induration around the site of injection at 48–72 h is the key outcome of the test. The DoH in its booklet *Immunization against Infectious Disease* (HMSO, 1992) provides instructions on the performance and interpretation of tuberculin tests.

• With the exception of infants up to the age of 3 months, all other individuals due to receive the BCG vaccine should first be tuberculin skin tested and found to be negative.

• The test should not be carried out within 3 weeks of receiving live viral vaccines, as they can suppress the test.

• Conditions which can suppress the reaction to tuberculin protein include viral infections (e.g. measles, rubella, glandular fever), sarcoidosis, Hodgkin's disease, immunosuppressing disease (including HIV) and corticosteroid therapy. If the skin test is negative, it should be repeated 2–3 weeks after clinical recovery.

• In individuals who have received the BCG vaccine it is not possible to determine whether a positive tuberculin skin test is caused by mycobacterial infection or by the BCG vaccination itself.

• Immunotherapy with BCG vaccine has been shown to be an effective treatment for superficial urine bladder carcinoma.

Vaccine availability

• Intradermal BCG Vaccine BP, Evans Medical Ltd, available in 10-dose and 50-dose vials with appropriate diluent.

• Percutaneous BCG Vaccine BP, Evans Medical Ltd, available in 10-multidose vials.

Any remaining vaccine after a vaccination session should be discarded, and if possible incinerated or treated with a disinfectant such as strong hypochlorite solution.

BCG vaccines are distributed to users by Farillon Ltd, on behalf of the DoH.

Storage. Between +2 and +8°C. *Do not freeze diluent.* Protect from light.

Tuberculosis infection

Almost all cases of human tuberculosis are caused by *Mycobacterium tuberculosis*, discovered by Robert Koch in 1882. It is an aerobic 'acid and alcohol-fast bacterium' (AAFB). The form of tuberculosis suffered by cattle, due to *M. bovis*, is rarely seen nowadays due to tuberculosis eradication programmes from farming practice (transmitted via ingestion of infected raw milk).

Transmission of tuberculosis is usually by inhalation of droplets from a patient with pulmonary tuberculosis; such droplets are sputum positive for the bacillus. The incubation period from infection to development of a positive reaction to tuberculin skin test is about 2–10 weeks. However, months or years may elapse from infection to development of disease and in most instances infection becomes dormant and never progresses to clinical disease. Reactivated tuberculosis is the most common clinical manifestation. Most tuberculosis cases are 'pulmonary', while 15% present with the 'extrapulmonary' form where any part of the body can be involved.

Factors that promote reactivation of tuberculosis are old age, malnourishment, concominant pulmonary disease, alcoholism, diabetes mellitus, gastric resection, corticosteroid therapy and immunosuppression including HIV disease. Risk groups for tuberculosis are patients with the above conditions, close contacts of smear positive patients, immigrants and people from ethnic minorities, the homeless and those living in poor, overcrowded conditions, older white people, and travellers (especially long-term) to areas of high prevalence.

In 1921, the French workers Albert Galmette and Camille Guérin of the Pasteur Institute produced the first human vaccine against tuberculosis. Half of the world's population has been injected with BCG vaccine since 1948 but its effectiveness differs, being more effective in some countries than in others. While in Britain it has been shown to be 70–80% effective, BCG has not been found to be so effective in some American trials and in India. Because of scepticism about its benefits, BCG is not routinely used in the USA; however, its cheapness, safety and ability to stimulate a long-term immune response has made it the most widely used vaccine in the world. While BCG may not always protect against tuberculosis, it may suppress the development of some of the more serious complications, particularly in children. For unknown reasons, BCG protection tends to decrease with age.

One-third of the world's population is infected with tubercle bacilli which may lie dormant for many years. WHO has reported between 7 000 000 and 8 000 000 new cases of tuberculosis every year (Fig. 1). Almost 3 000 000 people die each year from tuberculosis (Fig. 2). The largest numbers of cases and the largest increases have recently been reported in South-East Asia and western Pacific regions. Some of these increases have undoubtedly been due to improved case finding and reporting. At any one time worldwide there are 20 000 000 sufferers and 5000 000 infectious cases.

Over the past three decades, deaths from tuberculosis in England and Wales have declined from 2168 in 1964 to 422 in 1991. It is important to note that most deaths in recent years have been among the elderly age group of the indigenous white population. During the same period, the total number of notifications of tuberculosis in England and Wales declined from 17 627 in 1964 to 5086 in 1987, and have subsequently increased slightly but steadily to 5861 in 1992 and 6052 in 1993.

UK notification rates for tuberculosis are 20–30 times higher in people of Indian subcontinental origin than in the indigenous Caucasian population, and still higher in immigrants who have arrived recently.

There are no recommendations in the USA for routine BCG

vaccination for prevention of tuberculosis. Efforts for such control are directed towards early identification and treatment of infected persons, preventive therapy with isoniazid and prevention of transmission to others.

Until 1985, the prevalence of tuberculosis was declining in the USA, but since then there has been a steady climb with an overall increase of 16% between 1985 and 1990. In some urban centres, the rise has been more marked. Frieden *et al*. (*New Engl J Med* 1993; 328: 521–6) reported a 132% increase in tuberculosis notifications between 1980 and 1990 in New York, mainly among the 25–44 year age group, immigrants and ethnic minorities. This has been attributed largely to the increase in tuberculosis among those infected with HIV or diagnosed as having acquired immune deficiency syndrome (AIDS) (Fig. 3), an increase in homelessness in inner-city areas, increases in alcohol and IV drug use and the recent emergence of multidrug resistant strains of *Mycobacterium tuberculosis*. These phenomenon are also seen in Asia, Africa and the Pacific. New York City now has three times as many new cases of tuberculosis as any other city in the USA. Due to great efforts, New York City saw a 15% fall in the number of new cases reported in 1993 — a drop from 3811 new cases in 1992 to 3235 in 1993.

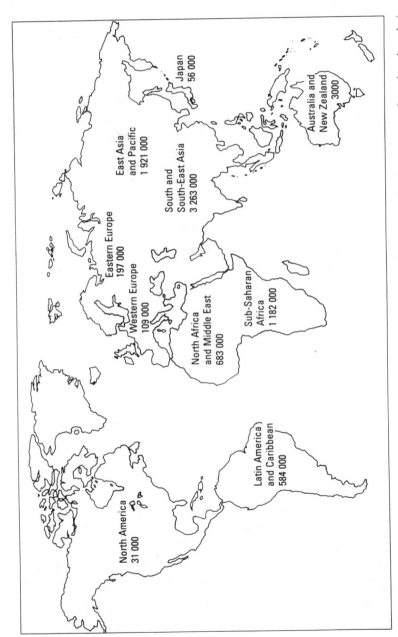

Fig. 1 Estimated incidence of tuberculosis cases in 1992; global total cases 8 000 000. Data reproduced with permission from the tuberculosis programme of the W.H.O.

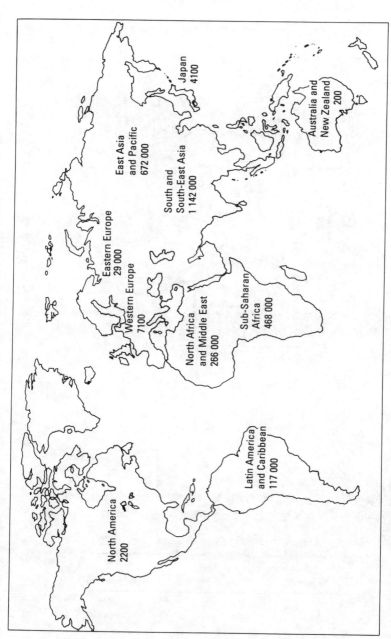

Fig. 2 Estimated mortality of tuberculosis in 1992; global total deaths 2 700 000. Data reproduced with permission from the tuberculosis programme of the WHO.

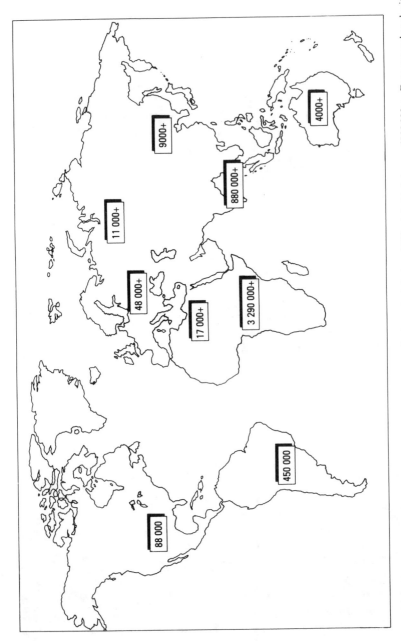

Fig. 3 Estimated global distribution of adults infected with HIV and tuberculosis in late 1993; global total cases 4800 000 + . Data reproduced with permission from the tuberculosis programme of the WHO.

Influenza

Contraindications to vaccination
● Acute febrile illness.
● Severe reaction to a previously administered flu vaccine.
● Anaphylactic hypersensitivity to hen's eggs.
● Severe hypersensitivity to neomycin and polymyxin (purified surface antigen vaccines: Fluvirin and Influvac).
● Severe hypersensitivity to thiomersal (disrupted virus vaccines: Fluzone, MFV-Ject, Fluarix).
● Pregnancy, unless there is a specific indication.

Possible side and adverse effects

Local reactions
Transient swelling, redness, pain and induration.

General reactions
Myalgia, malaise and fever for 1–2 days, beginning a few hours after vaccination. Neurological and anaphylactic reactions are very rare.

The vaccine
It is made from egg-grown viruses that are inactivated and highly purified. The vaccine is trivalent and contains two type A strains (H1N1 and H3N2) and one type B strain, representing the most recent influenza viruses circulating in the world. The types are recommended annually (in February) by WHO and the UK Joint Committee on Vaccinations and Immunisations Advisory Group. Their recommendations are based on the prevailing isolates received from an international network of laboratories.

Two types of vaccines of similar immunogenicity and side effects are currently available:
● Purified surface antigen vaccines (Fluvirin, Influvac): activated whole virus vaccine, prepared from purified virus particles. They are licensed for use in children from 4 years of age.
● Disrupted virus vaccine-split virion (Fluzone, MFV-Ject, Fluarix):

prepared by the additional step of disrupting the lipid-containing membrane of the virus. They are licensed for use in children from 6 months of age.

Administration

● Children who may not have been previously infected or who have not received the flu vaccine in the past 4 years (unprimed), require two doses of the vaccine, 4–6 weeks apart (Table 25).

● Flu vaccine should be given by IM or deep SC injection. The deltoid muscle is the recommended site for adults, the anterolateral thigh for children. In adults and especially elderly patients, the left arm should be avoided because of the possibility that left upper limb pain experienced may be attributed to the flu vaccine, when in fact this may be a symptom of myocardial ischaemia/infarction.

● Allow the vaccine to reach room temperature before injecting.

● The vaccine is effective if given 1 month (but at least 10 days) before exposure to the virus is anticipated. The UK flu vaccination programmes usually start in October.

● Clinical effectiveness in adults is about 70–80%. In elderly patients effectiveness can be less, nonetheless the vaccine's ameliorating effects and the ability to decrease the incidence and severity of complications

Table 25 Administration specifications for influenza vaccines

	Age	Dose (ml)	Previously unprimed
Purified surface antigen vaccines: Fluvirin, Influvac	4–13 years	0.5	Second dose 0.5 ml 4–6 weeks after first
	Over 13 years and adults	0.5	—
Disrupted (split) virus vaccines			
Fluzone, MFV-Ject	6–35 months	0.25	Second dose 0.25 ml 4–6 weeks after first
	3–12 years	0.5	Second dose 0.5 ml 4–6 weeks after first
	13 years and over, adults	0.5	—
Fluarix	6–71 months	0.25	Second dose 0.25 ml 4–6 weeks after first
	Over 6 years and adults	0.5	—

arising from influenza infection are very important, especially for elderly patients and those with chronic conditions.

● Flu vaccine can alter the hepatic clearance of several commonly used drugs, among them warfarin, phenytoin and theophylline. These changes do not seem to be clinically significant, nonetheless, the GP should be alert to this possibility.

● Revaccination each year should take place with the currently recommended vaccine and any unused vaccines from the previous year should not be given.

● Ensure that the practice has a yearly flu vaccination programme in place which includes the recall of high-risk patients for revaccination.

● Some elderly patients have bad memories of flu vaccination. It should be emphasized to them that the inactivated virus vaccines currently available are safe and virtually non-reactogenic. This is in contrast with live attenuated vaccines obtained prior to 1966, when 'having the vaccine was virtually as bad as having the disease'.

● The DoH's Chief Medical Officer writes to GPs yearly, giving advice on the recommendations for flu immunization for 'at-risk' patients. According to the DoH, groups at an increased risk for influenza-related complications and mortality are patients with:

(a) chronic respiratory disease, including asthma;

(b) chronic heart disease;

(c) chronic renal disease;

(d) diabetes mellitus and other endocrine disorders;

(e) immunosupression due to disease or treatment;

(f) residents of nursing homes and other chronic care facilities.

The DoH does not recommend routine immunization of fit children and adults, including health-care and other key workers such as home-care staff, district nurses, household members of high-risk persons, but leaves the final decision as to who should be offered immunization to the patient's medical practitioner.

● In the USA, yearly routine influenza immunization for healthy persons 65 years of age and over is recommended. Given the fact that 80–90% of influenza-associated excess mortality occurs among those aged over 65, and the increasing numbers of elderly persons, the impact of influenza in the UK is likely to increase unless we follow the American guidelines and immunize all elderly people over 65 years of age.

● Inactivated (killed) influenza vaccine does not cause influenza neither does it protect from other organisms that may cause respiratory and generalized infections during the influenza season. The expectations of patients, therefore, may differ from what the vaccine can deliver and they should be warned about this.

Vaccine availability

- Fluvirin, Evans Medical Ltd.
- Influvac, Duphar Laboratories Ltd.
- Fluzone, Servier Laboratories Ltd.
- MFV-Ject, Merieux UK Ltd.
- Fluarix, SmithKline Beecham Pharmaceuticals.

All available in single-dose 0.5 ml prefilled syringes. Shake before use.

Storage. Between +2 and +8°C. *Do not freeze.* Protect from light.

Influenza infection

In 15th century Florence, the influence (*influenza*) of the stars on the planets was thought to be the cause of this short febrile illness. In 1931, influenza virus type A was isolated from pigs and 2 years later from humans; type B was isolated in 1940 and type C in 1947.

Influenza A is the most important flu virus in humans and has been the cause of many epidemics and pandemics such as the Spanish flu in 1918, Asian flu in 1957, Hong Kong flu in 1968 and Red flu in 1977. The 1989 influenza epidemic was the worst to have hit England and Wales since 1976 and was most probably due to type A. During the epidemic, there were almost 22 000 more deaths than would be expected for that time of the year (only 10% of them were attributed to influenza on death certificates, and a further 5260 to pneumonia). Of these excess deaths, 60% were in women and more than 80% were people aged over 75. Every year we expect to see 3000–4000 deaths in the UK due to influenza, with incidence rising during epidemics.

Influenza A viruses are classified into subtypes on the basis of their two surface antigens, haemagglutinin (H) and neuraminidase (N). The human disease is caused by three H (H1, H2, H3) and two N (N1, N2) antigenic subtypes. Both antigens change with time (antigenic drift) so that previous infection or immunization becomes ineffective. Occasionally, there is a major change in the surface antigens (antigenic shift). Such antigenic variations also occur with influenza B viruses, although less frequently.

Influenza virus infection does not stimulate permanent immunity to reinfection with the same subtype of virus because of the new emerging variants. The same will apply to immunity acquired by vaccines which is even less effective. Protection from vaccination lasts for about 1 year. There is, therefore, a need for annual immunization in order to provide continuing protection.

Presentation

Influenza is an acute viral disease of the respiratory tract, affecting all ages. It presents with sudden onset pyrexia, headaches, chills and myalgia. A dry cough can follow with a sore throat and malaise. In mild to moderate cases it is a self-limiting disease lasting 2–7 days. In more severe cases, the virus can invade the lungs (primary viral pneumonia) or contribute to a secondary bacterial lung infection. It can be complicated by acute exacerbations of chronic respiratory disease or acute myo- carditis and may have neurological effects. Most at risk are patients who, because of their age or underlying health problems, are unlikely to cope with the disease.

There is some evidence that influenza A infection may be associated with fetal or perinatal mortality. Large epidemiological studies are necessary to confirm this association. Nonetheless GPs should be aware of the possibility of influenza A infection adversely influencing fetal survival.

Treatment

Physical rest, fluids and paracetamol are important. The only specific therapy available for influenza A virus is amantadine hydrochloride (Symmetrel); it is ineffective against type B virus. It prevents viral penetration of the cell membrane and has no direct viricidal action. It does not interfere with antibody production, whether from the vaccine or an actual infection.

Although it is as effective (60–80%) as influenza virus vaccine in preventing influenza A virus, it is not a substitute for annual immuni- zation of groups 'at risk'.

The DoH recommends amantadine during an outbreak of influenza A in the following circumstances, although it warns that indiscriminate use of amantadine could lead to viral resistance:

● for unimmunized patients 'at risk' for 2 weeks while the vaccine takes effect;

● for patients 'at risk' in whom immunization is contraindicated for the duration of the outbreak;

● for health-care workers and other key personnel to prevent disrup- tion of services during an epidemic.

The recommended dose is 100 mg daily. Adverse reactions occur in 5–20% of patients and include nausea, anorexia, lightheadedness, insomnia, headaches, restlessness, anxiety, difficulty in concentration and even depression. Epileptic fits may occasionally occur, mainly in elderly patients taking more than 100 mg a day.

Practice immunization programme

In the UK only 10–20% of those people considered to be 'at risk' do in fact receive the vaccine. A much greater effort to target these people is, therefore, needed by the members of the primary health-care team. All patients classified by the DoH as 'at risk' should be vaccinated if they agree. In addition, the practice may decide to extend the flu immunization programme to other patients, such as the over 60s.

The practice morbidity data, the age–sex register and the computerized repeat prescription system will be necessary. The practice can post invitations or attach them to the repeat prescriptions. As influenza activity is rarely significant before the end of November, the best time to start the immunization programme is October/November.

Experience from previous years and practice data should give an idea of the number of doses of flu vaccine needed.

Although there is no item-of-service fee payable for immunizing patients against flu, the practice can cover its expenses and even make a profit by buying and dispensing the vaccine under paragraph 44.5 of the *Statement of Fees and Allowances* (see p. 171). The practice profit depends to a great extent on the discount obtainable when buying directly from the manufacturers or wholesalers.

Influenza is a highly infectious disease that spreads rapidly in the community, especially in institutions. Epidemics occur in an unpredictable manner. Quite a number of patients tend to think of influenza as a relatively mild disease because it is confused with the common cold and other types of respiratory tract infections. In fact, influenza is a potentially lethal condition, especially in at-risk patients and elderly patients, and preventing it is an important community task for the GP.

Pneumococcal infection

Contraindications to vaccination

- Acute febrile illness.
- Severe reaction to a previously administered dose of the vaccine.
- Children under 2 years of age — the vaccine has limited immunogenicity (not effective) in these children.
- Pregnancy — it is not known whether the vaccine can cause fetal harm. If it is decided to immunize a pregnant woman with high-risk conditions such as cardiopulmonary or sickle cell disease, and it is not possible to vaccinate before pregnancy, it is advisable to wait until after the first trimester.
- Revaccination within 3 years — high risk of adverse reactions.
- The vaccine should be avoided during chemotherapy or radiotherapy and less than 10 days prior to commencement of such therapy because the antibody response is poor. Vaccination could be considered 3 months after discontinuation of chemotherapy.

Possible side and adverse effects

Local reactions
Swelling, redness, pain and occasionally induration.

General reactions
Fever and myalgia in less than 1% of vaccinees. Very rarely neurological disorders including Guillain–Barré syndrome, glomerulonephritis, relapse of thrombocytopenia in patients with idiopathic thrombocytopenic purpura, and anaphylactic reaction. Revaccination within 3–5 years or vaccination of individuals that have previously received the 14-valent pneumococcal vaccine may be associated with increased risk of reactions (because of high levels of circulating antibodies).

The vaccine
The 23-valent pneumococcal vaccine contains purified, capsular polysaccharide antigens of 23 pneumococcal serotypes responsible for 85–90% of bacteraemic infections. It has replaced the 14-valent vaccine.

The 23-valent vaccine contains 25 µg of each capsular polysaccharide antigen (the 14-valent vaccine contained 50 µg of each antigen). Following vaccination well over 80% of healthy adults will develop a good antibody response that will decline over the next few years (average protective level 7–10 years). Among elderly or asplenic patients this decline starts earlier so that protective antibody levels may not be present 6 or more years after vaccination. Immunosuppressed patients and young children respond less well to the vaccine.

Administration

- Protective antibody levels usually develop by the third week following vaccination. The overall protective efficacy of the vaccine is probably 65–70%. It is less effective in those who are immunocompromised.
- Boosters are not normally recommended other than for high-risk patients (see below) after 5–10 years. The presence of high pneumococcal antibody levels at the time of administration of a booster is associated with higher risk of local and general reactions. If in doubt, measure the specific antibody level. Revaccination with 23-valent vaccine is recommended for high-risk individuals who have received the 14-valent pneumococcal vaccine more than 6 years previously.
- When elective splenectomy or chemotherapy/radiotherapy is planned, the vaccine should be given approximately 2 or more weeks before the procedure. Ideally, enough time should be available before the procedure for measurement of specific antibody levels after vaccination that will show whether the patient has responded to the vaccination.
- Patients who require penicillin or other antibiotics for prophylaxis against pneumococcal infection should not discontinue their treatment after vaccination.

Table 26 Administration specifications for pneumococcal vaccine

Age	Dose (ml)	Route	Boosters
Adults	0.5	SC/IM Deltoid	5–10 years for high-risk persons
Children over 2 years	0.5	Anterolateral thigh	

● The vaccine is effective in preventing severe pneumococcal infections such as pneumonia or meningitis, but it gives no protection against more common infections where *Pneumococcus* can be implicated such as otitis media or exacerbations of chronic bronchitis. There are 84 known capsular pneumococcal serotypes (not all equally pathogenic) and only 23 serotypes are contained in the vaccine.

● *Indications:* in the UK, the DoH recommends pneumococcal vaccination for anybody over 2 years of age in whom pneumococcal infection is likely to be more common and/or dangerous (*Immunization against Infectious Disease*, HMSO, 1992). In particular the DoH recommends the vaccine for those with:

(a) homozygous sickle cell disease;

(b) asplenia or severe dysfunction of the spleen;

(c) chronic renal disease or nephrotic syndrome;

(d) immunodeficiency or immunosuppression due to disease or treatment, including HIV infection at all stages;

(e) chronic heart, lung and liver disease including cirrhosis; and

(f) diabetes mellitus.

● Advanced age is not included in the DoH recommendations, contrary to the advice of WHO and recommendations in the USA. In one study (*Lancet* 1992; 340: 1036–7) only one in three patients over 65 years of age with pneumococcal infection had risk factors that would have made them eligible for immunization under the UK recommendations. Several case–control studies have shown the efficacy of pneumococcal vaccine for selected elderly populations, both healthy and with co-existing disease.

● The DoH advises performing opportunistic pneumococcal immunization on 'at-risk' unimmunized patients at routine GP or hospital consultations, at discharge after hospital admission or when immunizing next time against influenza (pneumococcal vaccine is given once only). The aim is to curb rising infection in the UK caused by growing antibiotic resistance.

Vaccine availability

Pneumovax II, Merck Sharp & Dohme Ltd and Merieux UK Ltd., available in a single-dose vial. No dilution or reconstitution is necessary. Inspect before injection (clear, colourless liquid without suspended particles).

Storage: Between +2° and 8°C. *Do not freeze.*

Pneumococcal infection

Streptococcus pneumoniae (the pneumococcus) is a lancet-shaped, Gram-positive diplococcus. Eighty-four pneumococcal serotypes have been identified. Certain serotypes are prevalent in adults and others are prevalent in children.

Pneumococcal infections are most common during the winter months. Many people (up to 50% of healthy individuals) carry the organism in their upper respiratory tract without symptoms. Transmission is from droplets of respiratory tract secretions, from person to person. The incubation period is 1–3 days.

The pneumococcus accounts for up to 75% of community-acquired pneumonia. It is common in elderly people, among whom it causes severe illness and up to 25% mortality, especially in patients who develop bacteraemia or meningitis. In one study (*Lancet* 1992; 340: 1036–7) the case/fatality ratio for patients over 65 years of age was 40%.

Patients at risk of severe pneumococcal infection are patients with renal and cardiac failure, chronic pulmonary or liver disease and diabetes mellitus.

At particular risk are patients with impaired immunological response to the pneumococcus, that is patients with splenic dysfunction or splenectomy, patients with sickle cell anaemia, Hodgkin's disease, congenital or acquired immunodeficiency (including HIV), nephrotic syndrome and organ transplantation.

Symptoms depend on the site of infection, therefore they can be those of pneumonia, empyema, meningitis, pericarditis, endocarditis, peritonitis, otitis media or arthritis.

The commonest manifestation of pneumococcal infection is pneumonia. The onset of illness is usually sudden, with fever, rigors, myalgia, weakness, anorexia, chest pain (from involvement of the pleura) and cough, initially non-productive but later purulent.

Pneumococcal pneumonia is estimated to affect 1 in 1000 adults each year — about 50 000 cases in the UK. The incidence is higher among the elderly and patients with asplenism, Hodgkin's disease, myeloma, cirrhosis, heart disease and renal failure. It has a mortality rate of 10–20%.

The annual incidence of pneumococcal meningitis in the UK is approximately two cases per 100 000 of the population — about 400 reported cases per annum. Mortality ranges between 5 and 30%, with more deaths in the very young and the very old.

Pneumococcal bacteraemia occurs in all age groups with incidence estimated at 20 per 100 000 population. Among persons over 65 the incidence is 50 per 100 000 and in children under 2 years it is 160 per 100 000. Mortality among high-risk patients is high and estimated to be over 40%.

Asplenia

Patients with surgical or functional asplenia (for example, sickle cell disease) have reduced clearance of encapsulated bacteria, such as the pneumococcus, from their blood stream. Overwhelming infection after splenectomy can follow, caused most often by *Streptococcus pneumoniae* and *Haemophilus influenza* type b. Before splenectomy, patients should receive pneumococcal, meningococcal A and C and *Haemophilus influenza* b vaccines (check that the child has not already received Hib) and seroconversion checked before the surgical procedure. If immunization was not performed before splenectomy it should be done after the operation.

Since pneumococcal antibody levels may decline rapidly in some high-risk groups, GPs should consider monitoring these antibody responses, perhaps annually (> 21 IU/ml). Some patients in fact may need reimmunization earlier than the recommended 5–10 years.

In children, the risk of infection after splenectomy is high enough to justify a tablet of phenoxymethylpenicillin (penicillin V 125 mg up to age 6 years, 250 mg from 6 years onwards) once or twice daily, at least until their 16th birthday. Patients allergic to penicillin should take erythromycin.

Ideally, post-splenectomy patients should take prophylactic penicillin for life. On the other hand not many patients are willing to comply. In adulthood, by 5 years after splenectomy the risks of overwhelming infection are much reduced, to the point that prophylaxis could then be reserved for only the most vulnerable (those with malignant haematological disease or immunosuppression).

Patients unwilling to take regular penicillin should be made aware of the risks and supplied with penicillin to take immediately at the onset of suggestive symptoms. Consider recommending a Medic-Alert bracelet.

Finally, asplenic patients should be warned that they should avoid animal bites, especially dog bites as they can transmit *Capnocytophage canimorsus* that can lead to septicaemia and death if not treated early and appropriately with penicillin. They should avoid blood-borne protozoal infection such as babesiosis (transmitted by ticks) and malaria — strict adherence to the appropriate prophylaxis for the area being visited by travellers and avoidance of mosquito bites are essential.

Notes

Hepatitis A

Contraindications to vaccination
- Acute febrile illness.
- Severe reaction to a previously administered dose of hepatitis A vaccine.
- Severe hypersensitivity to any components of the vaccine such as aluminium hydroxide, phenoxyethanol and neomycin.
- Pregnancy and lactation, unless there is a definite risk of hepatitis A infection to the mother.
- Children under 1 year of age — the vaccine has not as yet been licensed for this age.

Possible side and adverse effects

Local reactions
Mild transient soreness, redness and induration.

General reactions
Flu-like symptoms such as fever, malaise, fatigue, headache, nausea and loss of appetite occur in up to 10% of vaccinees, lasting for 24–48 h. Elevation of liver enzymes has been reported.

The incidence of adverse effects, although mild, decrease with successive vaccine doses.

The vaccine
The vaccine available in the UK is formaldehyde-inactivated, prepared from the HM175 strain of hepatitis A virus (HAV) grown in human diploid cells. It is available as suspension, with each 1 ml containing 1440 enzyme-linked immunoadsorbent assayed (ELISA) units of HAV protein for adults, and 360 ELISA units in 0.5 ml for children. The vaccine is adsorbed on aluminium hydroxide and phenoxyethanol is used as a preservative. It contains traces of neomycin.

Administration

• The primary course of immunization for children consists of two doses, 2–4 weeks apart. Adults receive only one dose of the 1 ml Monodose vaccine. After the primary course the seroconversion rate is near 100% and provides anti-HAV antibodies for at least 1 year. A booster dose given at 6–12 months after the primary course will extend immunity to an estimated 10-year period (Table 27).

Table 27 Administration specifications for hepatitis A vaccine

Age	Dose (ml)	Route	Primary course	Reinforcing dose	Booster
1–15 years	0.5 (Junior)	IM	Two doses, 2–4 weeks apart	After 6–12 months	Every 10 years
Adults	1 (Monodose)	IM	One dose	After 6–12 months	Every 10 years

• Adults who have started a course of hepatitis A vaccine at the previously available adult dose of 720 ELISA units/ml should complete both the primary course and booster at this dosage.
• The prefilled syringe should be shaken well before use and the vaccine given IM, except in the case of patients with severe bleeding diathesis (i.e. haemophiliacs) in whom the SC route may be considered.
• The deltoid muscle is the recommended site of injection. The gluteal region should not be used because vaccine efficacy may be reduced.
• The minimum protective antibody concentration is 10 mIU/ml. The levels of antibody produced by the primary course and reinforcing dose are similar to those seen after natural HAV infection, and 100–300 times the level seen after a protective dose of HNIG.
• Adequate antibody titres may not be obtained after the primary course in patients on haemodialysis or with impaired immune systems. Such patients may require additional doses of the vaccine.
• The vaccine may be ineffective if given during the presence of hepatitis A infection (incubation time 15–40 days).
• Serotesting for anti-HAV IgG prior to vaccine administration may be worthwhile for those aged 50 years and over, or for individuals who were born and brought up in areas of high or intermediate HAV endemicity, or who have a history of jaundice. Some individuals of

ethnic minorities born in the UK may not be immune to HAV; older generations born overseas are more likely to be immune.

● Travellers, for whom hepatitis A vaccine might be indicated, who are due to travel in less than 2 weeks, may be given the first dose of vaccine if a child, or the Monodose if adult, in addition to HNIG (at different sites) and the course of vaccine completed on their return. In this case, seroconversion is not affected although the antibody titre will be lower.

● Following the primary course, protection is conferred within 2–4 weeks.

● HNIG, given before departure, cannot provide protection for travellers staying abroad for over 5 months. Early vaccination not only protects the traveller but removes the need to carry lyophilized immunoglobulin for repeat doses in countries with no reliable source of refrigerated HNIG.

● All recipients of clotting factors derived from plasma pools should be tested for antibodies to hepatitis A and, if found to be susceptible, offered a course of the inactivated hepatitis A vaccine. In such cases routine post-vaccination seroconversion testing is not necessary unless the recipient is known to be anti-HIV positive.

● Booster doses are important in order to avoid the possibility of converting a largely asymptomatic childhood disease into a symptomatic adult disease.

● GPs or practice nurses may be faced with a situation where more than 1 and less than 5 months have elapsed since the first dose was given to a child. In this case the second dose should be given, and the third (reinforcing) dose anytime between 6 and 12 months after the first dose (if the second dose is very late it may be better to give the third dose at 12 months). If more than 5 months have elapsed since the first dose, the whole course should be repeated.

Vaccine availability

Havrix Monodose Vaccine and Havrix Junior Vaccine, SmithKline Beecham Pharmaceuticals, available in prefilled syringes containing 0.5 ml (Havrix Junior Vaccine) and 1 ml (Havrix Monodose Vaccine) suspension in packs of one and 10.

Storage: Between +2 and +8°C. *Do not freeze.* Do not dilute. Protect from light. Shelf life of 2 years.

Human normal immunoglobulin

HNIG is prepared from plasma of at least 1000 blood donors. Serum proteins are separated and concentrated so that the solution contains 100–800 g/l of human plasma protein of which not less than 90% is IgG fraction.

There has been concern that falling prevalence of HAV infection in the UK general population might lead to HNIG not containing adequate levels of anti-HAV antibody. There have been no reported incidents where HNIG has failed to control outbreaks and it is known that even low levels (10 mlU/ml) of neutralizing antibody are enough to prevent infection. Nonetheless, there may soon be a need to use plasma from donors in high endemicity areas for the preparation of HNIG.

Each plasma donation and the final product is tested by validated procedures and found non-reactive for hepatitis B surface antigen and antibodies to HIV.

HNIG may be given simultaneously and at different sites with inactivated hepatitis A vaccine. It does not affect the seroconversion rate although the antibody levels achieved may be reduced.

When used for pre-exposure prophylaxis, it offers short-term protection (up to 5 months) against HAV infection, depending on the dose given. Travellers staying abroad in 'at-risk' areas for over 5 months have the option of carrying with them lyophilized immunoglobulin for repeated doses, provided it can be stored during travel at temperatures between +2 and +25°C.

Administation of HNIG early in the incubation stage of hepatitis A infection can prevent or attenuate the illness, but may not prevent virus excretion. Post-exposure HNIG prophylaxis is usually given to close contacts of patients with hepatitis A infection.

Before administration of HNIG, where practicable, serotesting for anti-HAV IgG may be worthwhile for those over 50 years of age, or for individuals who were born and brought up in areas of high or intermediate endemicity or who have a history of jaundice.

Contraindications to HNIG

● Severe reaction to a previously administered dose of HNIG.

● Within 3 weeks of administration of a live virus vaccine (measles, mumps, rubella, oral poliomyelitis) but not yellow fever as HNIG obtained in the UK is unlikely to contain antibody to yellow fever virus. If HNIG has been administered first, the live virus vaccines (except yellow fever) should not normally be given for 3 months. This contra-

Table 28 HNIG (with or without simultaneous administration of hepatitis A vaccine) should be considered in the following circumstances

Travellers	To intermediate or high endemicity areas, who are non-immune
Contacts	Of patients with hepatitis A infection. This group includes not only household contacts but also household visitors — kissing contacts and those who have eaten food prepared by the patient. Contacts in child day-care centres in order to protect adult staff — children are likely to have a mild to subclinical infection
Outbreaks	In institutions, closed communities and schools (children — although many of them would have been infected by the time HNIG is given — teachers and staff)
Newborn	Of a mother jaundiced at the time of delivery

indication may be ignored, especially as regards OPV when given to travellers with insufficient time for full immunization — consider co-administration of hepatitis A vaccine.

● Pregnancy, unless there is a risk of hepatitis A infection to the mother. There is inadequate evidence of safety in pregnancy, but HNIG has been widely used for many years without apparent adverse consequences.

Possible side and adverse effects

Local reactions Short-term discomfort at the injection site.

General reactions Very rarely anaphylactic reaction mainly in patients with hypoglobulinaemia, who have antibodies to IgA, or in patients who have had atypical reaction to blood transfusion or treatment with plasma derivates.

Administration

HNIG is administered as a single dose strictly IM. It must not be given IV since it may cause severe reaction. Recommendations and doses given in Table 29 refer to weight (mg) or volume (ml) of a 16% solution.

HNIG preparations should be stored in a refrigerator at between +2 and +8°C. The lyophilized form should be stored at temperatures of between +2 to +25°C.

HNIG

● Bio Products Laboratory.

Table 29 Dosage of HNIG — hepatitis A

Age	Low dose for 2 months travel	High dose for 3–5 months travel and for contacts
Under 10 years	125 mg	250 mg
10 years and over	250 mg	500 mg
All ages	0.02–0.04 ml/kg bodyweight	0.06–1.12 ml/kg bodyweight

- Kabiglobulin, Pharmacia, available in 2 and 5 ml ampoules.
- Gammabulin liquid, Immuno Ltd, available in 2, 5 and 10 ml ampoules; Gammabulin lyophilized 320 mg powder.
- Blood Transfusion Service, Scotland.
- The Laboratories, Belfast City Hospital.

Hepatitis A infection

HAV causes a spectrum of infection ranging from silent or subclinical infection, to clinical hepatitis with or without jaundice, to fulminant disease and death (mortality rate in excess of 2% in the over 40 age group). Asymptomatic disease is common in children and the severity tends to increase with age.

It is transmitted by the faecal–oral route and spreads mainly by person-to-person contact. Common source outbreaks may occur as a result of faecal contamination of food and drinking or coastal water. Sexual practice most likely to spread HAV is oral–anal contact. Recipients of clotting factors derived from plasma pools occasionally contract the disease. Transmission by blood transfusion is rare. On rare occasions infection has been contracted from non-human primates living in captivity and having had previous contact with man.

The disease is highly contagious because large numbers of viruses are shed during the long incubation period of the disease (15–40 days). It is also related to poor housing conditions with poor hygiene and sanitary conditions.

In most developing countries, infection by HAV is usually acquired subclinically in childhood but, as standards of hygiene and sanitation improve, children escape early infection only to be infected clinically and in large numbers as young adults. The largest ever recorded outbreak of hepatitis A infection occurred in Shanghai, China in 1988 and was attributed to the consumption of sewage-contaminated clams. More

Table 30 Risk groups for hepatitis A infection

Travellers	To areas of intermediate or high endemicity, therefore, non-immune travellers to countries outside northern and western Europe, North America, Australia, New Zealand and Japan. This group includes holiday and business travellers, airline personnel, foreign aid workers, missionaries, professionals working abroad, armed forces/diplomatic personnel and immigrants visiting country of origin
Occupations	Such as sewage workers, food handlers and food packagers, health-care workers particularly in paediatric specialities, child day-care staff at residential institutions for the mentally and physically handicapped where standards of personal hygiene are poor, and military personnel
Persons	Abusing drugs parenterally, male homosexuals, family members and close contacts of patients infected with HAV, carers of people whose personal hygiene may be poor, eating raw shellfish, living in poor housing conditions with poor standards of hygiene and sanitation, recipients of clotting factors derived from plasma pools

than 300 000 clinical cases of hepatitis A infection were reported, mostly in persons aged between 20 and 29. Before the outbreak, two-thirds of the population under 30 were susceptible.

Northern western Europe is an area of low endemicity. Spain, southern Italy and Greece are considered to be areas of intermediate endemicity while Turkey, and east and south Mediterreanean countries are areas of high endemicity (Fig. 4).

Most of the UK cases (over 80%) are contracted in the UK. In 1969, 21 000 cases of hepatitis A were notified in England; in 1982, 4000 cases; in 1991, 7000 cases and in the first 3 months of 1992, 2000 cases. Hepatitis A is a notifiable disease. About 1 400 000 cases are reported worldwide every year. The true incidence of course is much higher.

In many newly developed and industrialized countries, the provision of clean water for drinking and washing, modern sewage disposal systems and greatly increased standards of personal hygiene have reduced HAV prevalence. Immunity to hepatitis A infection within

Table 31 Markers of hepatitis A virus infection

Anti-HAV IgM	Indicates recent onset of HAV infection and persists for about 10 weeks
Anti-HAV IgG	Indicates past infection and immunity to HAV. It can be detected in serum, urine and saliva of infected individuals
Carrier state	Does not exist (but up to 10% of cases may relapse)

these populations is, therefore, falling leaving a growing pool of susceptible people. HAV continues to persist, putting non-immune people at risk.

At high risk are non-immune travellers and workers at 'high-risk' jobs. Regular passive immunization (with HNIG) against HAV is an impracticable preventive measure. Active immunization by vaccination offers long-term immunity.

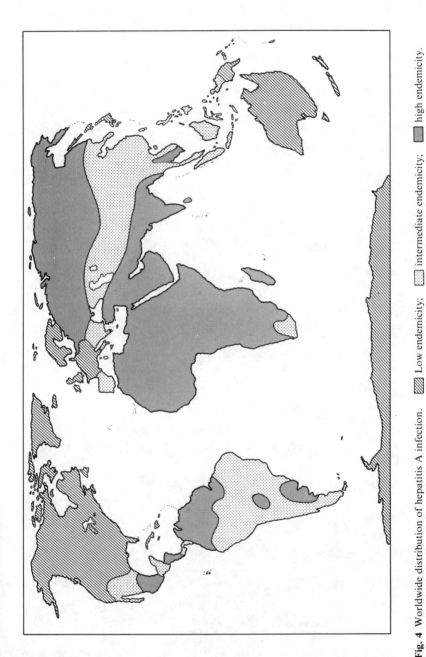

Fig. 4 Worldwide distribution of hepatitis A infection. ▨ Low endemicity; ▨ intermediate endemicity; ▨ high endemicity.

Notes

Hepatitis B

Contraindications to vaccination
- Acute febrile illness.
- Severe reaction to a previously administered dose of hepatitis B recombinant yeast vaccine.
- Severe hypersensitivity to aluminium or thiomersal.
- Pregnancy, unless there is a definite risk of hepatitis B to the mother or she is in a high-risk category.

Possible side and adverse effects

Local reactions
Mild transient soreness, erythema, swelling and induration in up to half of vaccinees. A persisting nodule can be formed if the vaccine is given ID.

General reactions
Pyrexia in the first 48 h, malaise, fatigue, headaches, nausea, dizziness, myalgia, vomiting, diarrhoea, arthralgia, abdominal pain and rashes including rarely erythema multiforme and urticaria. Neurological complications are very rare.

The inactive ingredient aluminium hydroxide is probably responsible for the local side effects. Some of the general side effects like urticaria may be due to another inactive ingredient, thiomersal.

The vaccine
The recombinant yeast vaccine is produced by yeast into which a plasmid containing the gene of the hepatitis B surface antigen (HBsAg) has been inserted. Each 1 ml of the vaccine contains 20 µg of HBsAg adsorbed on aluminium hydroxide adjuvant. Thiomersal is used as a preservative.

The hepatitis B carrier plasma derived vaccine is no longer available in the UK. Individuals immunized with this vaccine in the past can receive boosters using the recombinant yeast vaccine.

Administration

● The vaccine should be given by IM injection except in patients with severe bleeding diathesis (i.e. haemophiliacs) in whom the SC or ID route may be considered. However, the vaccine is only licensed for IM route as its administration by any other route is not often associated with an effective antibody response (dose: 2 µg/0.1 ml, ID route).

● The deltoid muscle is the preferred site of injection in adults and the anterolateral thigh in infants and younger children. The gluteal region should not be used because vaccine efficacy may be reduced.

● Shake the vial before withdrawing the vaccine suspension — once shaken, the vaccine is slightly opaque.

● The immunization regime consists of three doses of vaccine, the second dose at 1 month and the third at 6 months after the initial dose (0, 1 and 6 months). Where more rapid immunization is required (i.e. following exposure to the virus or travel), the third dose may be given at 2 months after the initial dose with a booster dose at 12 months (0, 1, 2 plus 12 months).

● The duration of protection and need for booster doses is not yet known precisely but it is thought to be in the order of 5–10 or more years.

● Protective antibody titres are achieved after the third dose of the 0, 1 and 6 month schedule and after the third dose of the 0, 1, 2 plus 12 month schedule (the booster dose at 12 months serves to prolong protection).

● Check antibody titres 6–8 weeks after completion of the primary course (three doses). Such a course induces seroconversion in 99% of healthy young adults with an adequate antibody response to the HBsAg (anti-HBs > 100 mIU/ml) in more than 90%, and in more than 95% of

Table 32 Administration specifications for hepatitis B vaccine

Age	Dose	Route	Primary immunization	Booster
0–12 years	10 µg (0.5 ml)	IM	0, 1, 6 months (accelerated course: 0, 1, 2 plus 12 months)	5–10 years
Adults	20 µg (1 ml)	IM		5–10 years
Immunocompromised and dialysis patients	20–40 µg (1–2 ml)	IM		5–10 years (check antibody level periodically)

infants, children and adolescents. A peak antibody concentration of 100 mIU/ml can be expected to fall significantly, even below 10 mIU/ml in about 5 years, which has been the basis for scheduling booster doses of hepatitis B vaccine.

● A good response to the vaccine is considered to be the achievement of anti-HBs level > 100 mIU/ml. Inadequate response ('no response') is a level of < 10 mIU/ml — these individuals make up 5–10% of those immunized.

● There is some evidence that protective immunity can still be present with antibody levels < 100 mIU/ml. It has also been suggested that immunity may persist even after antibody levels have fallen to undetectable levels. In this case, it is suggested that one has to rely on the immunological memory to protect. The current advice is that individuals who remain at high risk of exposure to hepatitis B virus (HBV) should have their antibody level determined periodically. If the anti-HBs level falls below 100 mIU/ml, the need for a booster dose should be considered.

● The administration of the vaccine to individuals known to be hepatitis B surface antigen, or antibody, positive is unnecessary as they are carriers and immune. Inadvertent vaccination would merely boost antibody levels. The vaccine is ineffective when given to patients with acute hepatitis B.

● The vaccine may be given to HIV positive individuals.

● The recombinant yeast hepatitis B vaccine may be given simultaneously with all other vaccines and immunoglobulins but a different syringe and site should be used. This vaccine cannot cause liver cancer as it contains only purified surface antigen. Recipients of this vaccine can donate blood starting 1 week after a dose.

● Hepatitis B vaccine protects also against hepatitis D (δ) as the latter only occurs in individuals infected with hepatitis B virus.

Table 33 Type of response to hepatitis B vaccine and the need for a booster dose

Type of response	Anti-HBs level (mIU/ml)	Booster dose recommendations
No response	Negative	Immediate or repeat course
Inadequate response (consider as no response)	< 10	Immediate or repeat course
Low response	10–100	6 months to 2 years
Good response	> 100	5–10 or more years

Table 34 Situations associated with low or no hepatitis B antibody response following hepatitis B vaccination

- 5% of normal individuals under the age of 40 years
- Increasing age (over 40 years)
- Male sex
- Chronic renal failure, renal dialysis
- Alcoholic liver disease, cirrhosis
- Obese individuals
- Cigarette smokers
- Infection with HIV (seroconversion in 50–70% of cases)
- Treatment with immunosuppressive or cytotoxic drugs
- Genetic predisposition (e.g. HLA-B8)
- Presence of hepatitis B infection (incubation time 45–160 days) at the time of vaccination — the vaccine may be ineffective
- Vaccine administered by route other than IM, and at other site than the deltoid in adults and the anterolateral thigh in children
- Incorrect vaccine storage, e.g. frozen, or vaccine out of date.

- Contacts of patients with acute hepatitis B should be passively immunized (see p. 106) and vaccinated simultaneously and at a different site.
- Acute exposure to infected blood should be treated by passive immunization with hepatitis B immunoglobulin (HBIg) and active immunization with hepatitis B vaccine or a booster dose if previously immunized, unless known to have adequate protection level (> 100 mIU/ml) of antibodies.
- Children born to mothers who are hepatitis Be antigen (HBeAg) and HBsAg positive are at greatest risk and best protected by being vaccinated (10 μg dose) at birth or as soon as possible thereafter, preferably within 12 h and not later than 48 h. At the same time HBIg (200 IU) should be given in a different syringe and at a different site. The course of vaccination should be continued according to the 0, 1 and 6 month schedule or the 0, 1, 2 plus 12 month rapid immunization schedule.
- Hepatitis B, as a sexually transmitted disease, is the only such disease we can prevent by immunization.

Vaccine availability
- Engerix B, SmithKline Beecham Pharmaceuticals, available in monodose vials containing 1 ml suspension in packs of one, three (OP) and 10.

Table 35 Risk groups for hepatitis B — recommendations for pre-exposure vaccination

Health-care workers	Doctors, dentists, nurses (especially in emergency wards and intensive care units); midwives; ancillary staff in contact with patient material; laboratory technicians handling blood; research workers at risk of contamination; blood bank personnel; drug dependency units and mental institution personnel; medical/dental/nursing students; dental hygienists and nurses; acupuncturists; health workers on secondment to work in high-risk areas abroad
Patients	Requiring frequent blood transfusions (e.g. thalassaemia major, leukaemia); haemophiliacs, patients on haemodialysis, renal transplants; mentally handicapped in institutions; babies born to mothers with acute or chronic hepatitis B
Persons	Abusing drugs parenterally; homosexual men; bisexual men; heterosexuals with multiple partners; prostitutes; inmates of long-term custodial institutions; carers, household and sexual contacts of patients with acute or chronic hepatitis B; immigrants from countries with high carrier rates
Emergency service and high-risk workers	Selected police, ambulance and rescue services; staff at custodial institutions; staff at institutions for the mentally handicapped; morticians and embalmers
Travellers	Long stay in high-risk hepatitis B areas; likely to require medical or dental procedures carried out in high-risk countries; tourists with sexual behaviour placing them at risk

● Engerix B Paediatric, available in monodose vials containing 0.5 ml suspension in packs of one.

Storage. Between $+2$ and $+8°$C. *Do not freeze.* Protect from light. Do not dilute. Shelf life of 3 years.

Human hepatitis B immunoglobulin

● Human hepatitis B immunoglobulin (HBIg) is prepared from plasma of donors who have been found to have suitably high titres of hepatitis B antibodies. Each plasma donation and the final product are tested by validated procedures and found non-reactive for antibodies to HIV (HIV-1).

● In the case of accidental exposure, allow the wound or cut to bleed and wash with soap and water. If the skin is contaminated, wash with soap and water. Rinse any eye splashes with water or sterile saline solution.

● Where immediate protection is required, such as after exposure to hepatitis B virus, HBIg and hepatitis B vaccine should be administered simultaneously, with separate syringes and into separate injection sites — HBIg does not inhibit the antibody response to hepatitis B vaccine. Individuals who are known to have received hepatitis B immunization in the past should be given a booster dose of vaccine, unless they are known to have adequate protective levels of antibody, i.e. anti-HBs > 100 mIU/ml.

● HBIg should be administered as soon as possible after exposure, preferably within 48 h, and not later than 1 week. A second dose of HBIg should be given 4 weeks later unless:

(a) there is evidence of past hepatitis B infection in the recipient's pre-HBIg blood sample;

(b) tests show that the HBsAg positive inoculum is anti-HBe positive (low risk of infectiousness); or

(c) hepatitis B vaccine was given at or about the time the first dose of HBIg was given.

● Newborn of mothers who had hepatitis B during pregnancy or early puerperium, or mothers who are surface antigen positive should receive active/passive immunization. Hepatitis B immunoglobulin should be given as soon as possible after birth, preferably within 12 h. Efficacy of HBIg given at 12–48 h is presumed but unproven. Hepatitis B vaccine should be given at the same time in a different syringe and at a different site. The second and third doses are given at 1 and 6 months after the first. If vaccine is not given in the first 12 h after birth, the first dose should be given within the first 7 days. If vaccine administration is delayed for as long as 3 months, a second dose of HBIg should be given.

● In up to 2% of cases, the passive/active immunization (HBIg/hepatitis B vaccine) is not effective. Infants should be serotested at 9 months of age or later (at least 1 month after the third vaccine dose), for surface antigen and antibody. If an infant is found to be surface antigen

Table 36 Hepatitis B immunoglobulin is recommended in these circumstances

---

● Accidental exposure to hepatitis B virus such as occurs when blood or other material containing surface antigen is inoculated, ingested or splashed onto mucous membranes or the conjunctivae. This is important for practice staff who perform invasive procedures and themselves fail to seroconvert

● Family contacts judged to be at high risk, and sexual contacts as well as carers of patients with acute hepatitis B

● Newborn of mothers with acute hepatitis B in pregnancy or early in the puerperium

● Newborn of mothers who are hepatitis B surface antigen positive, particularly if e antigen is detectable. Such infants rarely display any symptoms but have a 70–90% chance of becoming chronic carriers

---

Table 37 Dosage of human hepatitis B immunoglobulin

Age		Dose IU
Newborn	IM soon after birth, within first 12 h. Give simultaneously hepatitis B vaccine (10 µg) in a separate syringe and at a different site	200
Children	Age 0–4 years	200
	Age 5–9 years	300
	Age > 10 years	500
Adults		500

and antibody negative, he or she should receive a fourth dose of vaccine and be retested 1 month later for antibody to HBsAg.

● HBIg is not appropriate for travellers to high-risk areas. Hepatitis B vaccination is more appropriate under these circumstances.

● HBIg is available in 2 ml ampoules (200 I U) and 5 ml ampoules (500 I U). It should be used as a single dose I M and must never be given I V.

Hepatitis B immunoglobulin availability

The DoH advises that supplies in the U K are limited and demands should be restricted to patients in whom there is clear indication for its use. It is available from the following places:

● Communicable Disease Surveillance Centres.
● Local public health laboratories.
● Bio Products Laboratory.
● Blood Transfusion Service, Scotland.
● Regional Virus Laboratory, Belfast.

Hepatitis B infection

● Hepatitis B virus (H B V) causes a spectrum of infection ranging from asymptomatic seroconversion to fulminant, fatal hepatitis. Its chronic complications include hepatic cirrhosis, necrosis, chronic active hepatitis and hepatocellular carcinoma.

● The major modes of hepatitis B virus transmission are contact with blood and through sexual activity. Apart from blood, it can be found in wound exudate, breast milk, semen, cervical secretions, vaginal fluid and saliva, although the latter is not an effective vehicle for transmission. The virus has been shown to survive in dried blood, outside the body, for at least 1 week in ambient conditions.

● The routes of infection for children and adults are different.

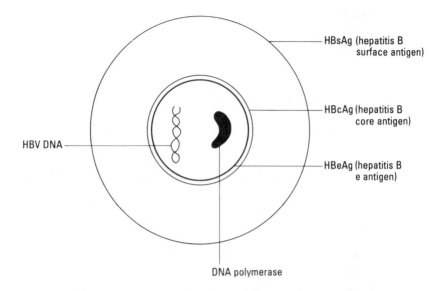

Fig. 5 Hepatitis B virus.

Children may acquire hepatitis B virus by vertical transmission (infection of the newborn from mother) or horizontal spread (via bites and cuts). The commonest modes of transmission in adults are sexual intercourse and percutaneous inoculation.

● Seroprevalence studies show that infection begins to increase between 12 and 18 years of age and steadily increases with advancing age thereafter. The hepatitis B virus is at least 100 times more infectious than HIV.

● The hepatitis B virus chronic carrier is defined as a person who is positive for surface antigen for 6 months or more. Approximately 5–10% of adults infected become chronic carriers. Of them, up to 25% will develop chronic active hepatitis which often leads to cirrhosis or hepatocellular carcinoma and death. Infants born to carrier mothers have a 70–90% chance of becoming chronic carriers.

● Infection with the hepatitis B virus results in the appearance of core antibody in the serum, and in most people this antibody will persist for many years indicating past infection. Those who become carriers of the hepatitis B virus will persistently test positive for surface antigen. Those who become immune will test positive for surface antibody.

● Immunization with hepatitis B vaccine results in seropositivity for surface antibody alone (anti-HBs positive).

Table 38 Serological markers for hepatitis B virus infection and immunity

Hepatitis B surface antigen	The first screening test — detection of carriers or acutely infected patients
Antibody to hepatitis B surface antigen	Indicates past infection or immunization and immunity
Hepatitis B e antigen	Indicates acute hepatitis or that the patient is a highly infectious chronic carrier
Antibody to hepatitis B e antigen	Indentifies hepatitis B surface antigen carriers with low risk of infectiousness
Antibody to hepatitis B core antigen	Identifies persons who have had hepatitis B infection in the past
IgM antibody to hepatitis B core antigen	Indicates acute or recent hepatitis B infection
Hepatitis B virus DNA	Indicates viral replication and high infectivity

- If the previously immunized person is found to be positive for core antibody it indicates that this person has previously acquired hepatitis B infection or it may coincide with acute clinical hepatitis. If in addition this person has persistent surface antigenaemia, he or she is at high risk of chronic hepatitis which can lead to cirrhosis and hepatocellular carcinoma.

- A successfully immunized person with persistent protective antibody to HBsAg (> 100 mIU/ml) when exposed to infection may become infected, as shown by anticore seroconversion, but this is rarely associated with acute hepatitis.

- Hepatitis B virus has infected millions of people worldwide. Globally, it is the ninth most common cause of death. About 300 000 000 people are chronically infected worldwide (about 5% of the earth's population). The average chronic carrier state can be as high as 20% in South-East Asia and as low as 0.1% in northern Europe.

- WHO estimates that 1000 000 people are infected with the virus each year. Of these about 90 000 will become chronically infected and 22 000 will eventually die from cirrhosis or hepatocellular carcinoma.

- The frequency of hepatitis B infection varies markedly in different parts of the world. Surface antigen endemicity below 2% is found in northern western Europe, the USA, southern Canada, Australia and New Zealand. In contrast, highly endemic areas (carrier rate between 8 and 20% — with some 'pockets' as high as 95%) are China, South-East Asia, most of Africa, the Arabian Peninsula, the Middle East, Alaska, most Pacific Islands and the Amazon Basin. In other parts of the world,

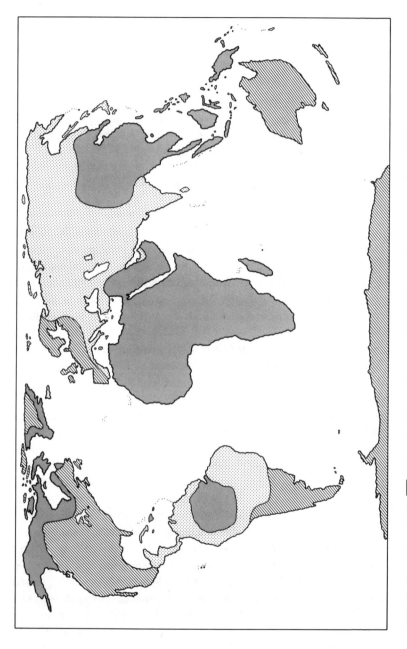

Fig. 6 Distribution of hepatitis B. ▨ High endemicity carrier rate > 8%; ▨ intermediate carrier rate 2–8%; ▨ low endemicity carrier rate ≤ 2%.

hepatitis B infection is moderately endemic with 2–7% of the population being carriers (Fig. 6).

● Over 30 countries (including the USA) have now opted to integrate hepatitis B into childhood immunization schedules. Mass immunization programmes have already been instituted in endemic areas such as China, Taiwan, Singapore, Gambia, Italy and some countries in the Arabian Peninsula.

● WHO advises that routine programmes of infant immunization against hepatitis B must be implemented by 1997, even in countries with low carrier rates such as the UK. Countries with carrier rates above 8% are advised to introduce routine hepatitis B immunization by 1995.

● Although the carrier state in the UK is below 2%, there are 'pockets' in the country where it exceeds this level. It is not as yet known when the DoH will be advising integration of hepatitis B immunization into the routine UK schedule of immunization, but it should be so by 1997.

● Hepatitis B infection can be eliminated by population education and immunization. It is estimated that if the UK was to now institute infant, adolescent and high-risk group immunization, the disease could be eliminated by the year 2015.

● Hepatitis B is a notifiable disease.

The United Kingdom Advisory Group on Hepatitis — guidelines for protecting health-care workers and patients from hepatitis B

These guidelines (Health Service Guidelines (93)40) were issued to UK health-care workers in August 1993. Their purpose is:

● to ensure that health-care workers who may be at risk of acquiring hepatitis B virus from patients are protected by immunization;

● to protect patients against the risk of acquiring hepatitis B virus from an HBeAg positive (highly infectious) health-care worker.

They recommend that:

● health-care workers who are HBeAg positive (highly infectious) must not carry out 'exposure prone procedures' in which there is a risk that injury to themselves could result in their blood contaminating a patient's open tissues;

● all health-care workers who perform 'exposure prone procedures' should be given the hepatitis B vaccine. Their level of seroconversion should be checked 2–4 months after the third dose. Those found to have antibody to surface antigen level < 10 mIU/ml, with their consent, should be tested for serological markers of past or current hepatitis B virus infection:

(a) those without markers of previous infection (anti-HBc negative, anti-HBs negative) may be at risk of hepatitis B infection. Their practice need not be restricted provided that occupational exposures are promptly reported and managed appropriately. Consider another course of vaccine and/or regular testing;

(b) those found to have naturally acquired immunity (anti-HBc positive, HBsAg negative) are not at risk of infection;

(c) those found to have current infection (HBsAg positive, anti-HBe positive) should have markers of infectivity checked. If e antigen positive: exclude from all 'exposure prone procedures' and refer for treatment and occupational advice. If e antigen negative, anti-HBe positive or negative: no need to change work practices.

These guidelines apply to all health-care workers, e.g. doctors, nurses, midwives, dentists, dental workers, medical and dental students, etc. They go further to point out that employers should make compliance with the guidance a condition of service for new staff appointed to posts that will involve 'exposure prone procedures', and should also ensure that locum or agency staff have complied with the guidance. Provider units should aim to vaccinate and check the immunity of all surgeons by mid-1994, and all staff involved in 'exposure prone procedures' by mid-1995.

Yellow fever

Contraindications to vaccination
● Acute febrile illness.
● Infants below the age of 9 months — infants under 4 months of age are more susceptible to adverse reactions of the vaccine (encephalitis) than older children and this risk is age-related. Consider vaccination of infants aged between 4 and 9 months only if travelling to an area of epidemic activity.
● Previous severe reaction to the vaccine.
● Anaphylactic hypersensitivity to neomycin, ploymyxin and hen's eggs.
● Pregnancy, although if a pregnant woman must travel to an area of high yellow fever risk, vaccination should be considered as the risk of infection may outweigh the small theoretical risk to the fetus from vaccination.
● Immunodeficiency and malignancy.
● HIV positive individuals whether asymptomatic or symptomatic.
● Within 3 weeks of administration of another live virus vaccine but may be administered simultaneously and at a different site. Within 3 weeks of administration of the live bacterial BCG.
● Give the cholera vaccine simultaneously or, better still, separate by 3 weeks as it may inhibit antibody response to both vaccines.
● Yellow fever vaccine can be given simultaneously with HNIG, which in the UK is unlikely to contain antibody to the yellow fever virus.

Possible side and adverse effects

Local reactions
Swelling, redness and pain lasting 2–5 days (5%).

General reactions
These are generally mild. Headaches, myalgia and low-grade fever in 5–10% of vaccinees, lasting 5–10 days after vaccination. Less than 0.2% will need to limit their activities. Rash, urticaria and jaundice are extremely rare. Encephalitis temporarily associated with vaccination

was reported (in the USA) in two cases out of more than 34 000 000 doses of the vaccine.

The vaccine
It is a live attenuated virus vaccine prepared from the 17D strain of yellow fever virus grown in chick embryos.

Administration
● The reconstituted vaccine should be given within an hour by deep SC injection. The dose is the same for all ages.

● It is recommended that apart from travellers, laboratory workers handling infected material should be immunized.

● The immunity, which probably lasts for life, is officially accepted for travel for 10 years starting from 10 days after primary immunization and immediately after a booster.

● For the purposes of international travel, the vaccine is administered only at yellow fever vaccination centres approved by the DoH. These centres meet stringent conditions regarding transportation, handling, storage, administration and documentation. They issue the International Certificate of Vaccination for Yellow Fever which is required for entry into or exit from some countries.

Table 39 Administration specifications for yellow fever vaccine

Dose (ml)	Route	Schedule	Booster
0.5	SC	Once only	Every 10 years (for travellers)

● The GP should supply an official letter of exemption to a patient who cannot, for medical reasons, receive the vaccine. However, this letter may not be accepted by certain countries, so it may be necessary to use this letter to obtain an official waiver stamped by the embassy of the countries to be travelled through or to. Otherwise, the traveller may risk quarantine, or sometimes vaccination at the border using needles of sometimes questionable sterility.

Vaccine availability
Yellow Fever Vaccine Live BP, Evans Medical Ltd, available as freeze-dried vaccine supplied to designated centres only, in packs of one and

five dose vials, with diluent. Available from DoH Yellow Fever Vaccination Centres only.

Storage: Between +2 and +8°C. *Do not freeze diluent.*

Yellow fever infection

The virus is believed to have originated in Africa and to have crossed the Atlantic by trading and slaving ships which may have introduced one of its important vectors, the mosquito *Aedes aegypti*. The first reported

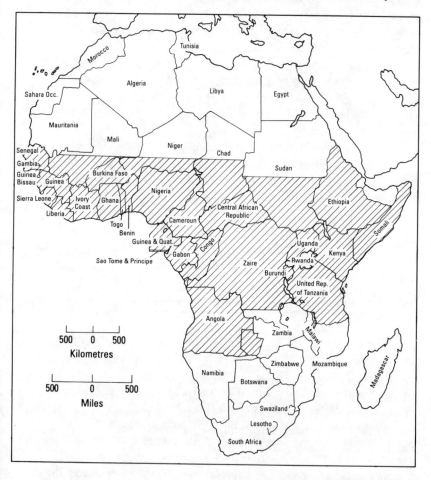

Fig. 7 Yellow fever endemic zone in Africa. ▨. Reproduced with permission from the WHO.

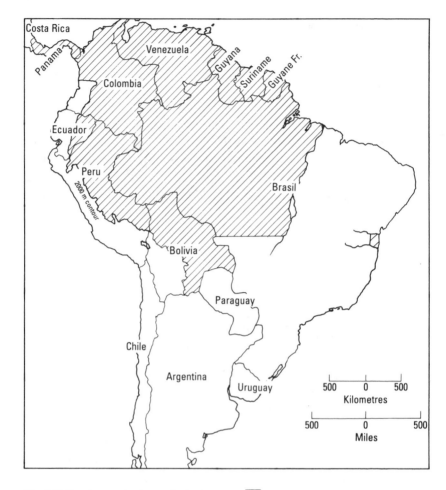

Fig. 8 Yellow fever endemic zone in the Americas. ▨ . Reproduced with permission from the WHO.

outbreak was in Barbados in 1647. It is today endemic in equatorial Africa and in parts of South America (Figs 7 and 8).

The main non-human host of the virus is the monkey and is transmitted to man via the bite of an infected mosquito. The incubation period is 2–5 days. Symptoms include vomiting, red tongue, swollen/ bleeding gums and congested conjunctivae. Jaundice appears in the convalescence period. The clinical presentation varies from a minor illness to a fulminating disease and death. It is still the most important cause of viral haemorrhagic disease in the endemic areas of Africa and South America.

Control of yellow fever is by eradicating the vectors, protection from mosquito bites and most importantly by immunization.

Notes

Typhoid

There are now three typhoid vaccines licensed in the U K. The two newer vaccines induce protection comparable to that induced by the killed whole-cell vaccine previously available. The added advantages are the reduction in side effects and route of administration.

Whole-cell typhoid vaccine

Contraindications to vaccination
● Acute febrile illness.
● Chronic illnesses — patients with chronic diseases such as multiple sclerosis, rheumatoid arthritis, diabetes and compensated cardiac conditions who are in remission may suffer a relapse as a result of an adverse reaction to vaccination with whole-cell vaccines (typhoid and cholera).
● Severe reaction to a previously administered dose of whole-cell typhoid vaccine.
● Children under 12 months of age because of the low incidence of typhoid, the mild course of the disease, and the risk of adverse reactions.
● Pregnancy is a relative contraindication and the vaccine should only be given if there is a clear risk of infection.

Possible side and adverse effects

Local reactions. Transient redness, swelling, pain and induration lasting from 1 to 2 days in up to a third of recipients.

General reactions. Myalgia, malaise, nausea, headaches and pyrexia for 1–2 days, beginning a few hours after vaccination. The incidence of systemic reactions is considerably reduced after ID administration, especially in the over 35s. Neurological and anaphylactic reactions very rarely occur.

The vaccine

The monovalent whole-cell vaccine contains 1000 000 000 heat-killed phenol-preserved *Salmonella typhi* organisms per millilitre.

Administration

● The first dose of the primary course is given IM or SC, while the second dose and boosters may be given by ID injection in order to minimize systemic reactions. Shake the bottle well to resuspend the vaccine before withdrawing the dose.

● In the case of urgent travel, one dose of the primary course may almost be as effective for a short period as two doses. The course can be completed on return.

● If longer than 3 years have elapsed since the primary course or a booster, a single dose is still sufficient.

● It confers 70–90% protection in recipients against typhoid.

Table 40 Administration specifications for whole-cell typhoid vaccine

Age	Primary course			Booster interval
	First dose	Time interval	Second dose and boosters	
Children 1–10 years	0.25 ml IM/SC	4–6 weeks	0.25 ml IM/SC or 0.1 ml ID	Every 3 years
Children over 10 years and adults	0.5 ml IM/SC	4–6 weeks	0.5 ml IM/SC or 0.1 ml ID	Every 3 years

Vaccine availability

Monovalent Typhoid Vaccine BP, Evans Medical Ltd, available in multidose vials of 1.5 ml — discard partly used vaccine vials.

Storage: Between +2 and +8°C. *Do not freeze.*

Typhim Vi vaccine

Contraindications to vaccination

- Acute febrile illness.
- Severe reaction to a previously administered dose of the vaccine.
- Children under 18 months of age may show a suboptimal response to the vaccine. The decision to vaccinate children under 18 months should be based upon the risk of exposure to typhoid.
- Pregnancy is a relative contraindication and the vaccine should only be given if there is a clear risk of infection.

Possible side and adverse effects

Local reactions. Swelling, redness and pain in 20% of recipients during the first 2–3 days after vaccination.

General reactions. Myalgia, malaise, nausea, headaches and pyrexia in approximately 3% of recipients.

The vaccine

It is a parenteral vaccine containing purified Vi polysaccharide antigen extracted from the bacterial capsule of *Salmonella typhi* strain Ty2. Vi antigen is believed to be important in inducing protective antibodies against typhoid. Each 0.5 ml dose contains 25 μg of this antigen.

Administration

- The vaccine should be given by deep SC or IM injection.
- Antibody seroconversion is seen in over 90% of vaccinees.
- It confers 60–80% protection against typhoid in recipients. Protection commences within 14 days from vaccination.

Table 41 Vaccination specifications for typhim Vi vaccine

Age	Primary course	Boosters
Adults and children over 18 months	0.5 ml SC/IM (single dose)	0.5 ml SC/IM every 3 years

Vaccine availability

Typhim Vi Vaccine, Merieux UK Ltd, available as a single-dose pre-filled syringe. Shake before use.

Storage: Between +2 and +8°C. *Do not freeze.*

Oral typhoid vaccine

Contraindications to vaccination

● Acute febrile illness.

● Acute gastrointestinal illness. Do not vaccinate while diarrhoea and vomiting persist.

● Severe reaction to a previously administered dose of the oral vaccine.

● Immunodeficiency and malignancy.

● HIV positive individuals whether asymptomatic or symptomatic.

● Pregnancy, unless the mother is at great risk of infection (it is not known whether the vaccine can cause fetal harm or whether it is passed in human milk).

● Children under 6 years of age — safety and efficacy have not as yet been established.

● Interactions include:

(a) sulphonamides and antibiotics — as they may be active against the vaccine strain causing inhibition of protective immune response;

(b) mefloquine for malarial chemoprophylaxis should not be taken on the same day — separate by at least 12 h; and

(c) oral polio vaccine should be separated from the oral typhoid vaccine by 2 weeks, until there is data about possible interaction in their gut replication.

● There is no need to separate the administration of the oral typhoid vaccine from other parenteral live vaccines or HNIG.

Possible side and adverse effects

Transient mild nausea, vomiting, abdominal cramps, diarrhoea and urticarial rash in less than 1% of vaccinees. In safety trials, adverse reactions occurred with equal frequency among groups receiving vaccine and placebo.

The vaccine

Each oral live vaccine capsule contains 2×10^9 organisms of the atte-nuated *Salmonella typhi* strain Ty21a in a lyophilized form.

Administration

● The vaccine capsule should be swallowed whole (do not chew) immediately after placing it in the mouth, with cold or lukewarm water (no warmer than 37°C), approximately 1 h before a meal.

Table 42 Administration specifications for oral typhoid vaccine

Age	Primary course			Boosters for frequent travel to endemic areas
	Dose	Frequency	Boosters	
Adults and children over 6 years	One capsule	On alternate days × three doses	Three-dose course every 3 years	Three-dose course annually

● The capsules must be kept refrigerated and all three doses must be taken to achieve maximum efficacy. In the USA four doses are used.

● Protection against typhoid commences approximately 7–10 days after completion of the three-dose course.

● In field trials in endemic areas with a three-dose alternate-day schedule the oral typhoid vaccine achieved protection in up to 96%. In a study amongst previously unexposed subjects with a multidose schedule (five to eight doses) 87% protection was achieved.

Vaccine availability
Vivotif Typhoid Live Oral Vaccine, Evans Medical Ltd. One pack comprises three enteric-coated capsules, each representing one dose. The blister containing the vaccine capsules should have an intact foil seal.

Storage: Between +2 and +8°C in a dry place, protected from light. It is important to stress to the patients who will self-administer the vaccine that it must be refrigerated.

Which vaccine?

None of the available vaccines are a substitute for close attention to personal, food and water hygiene.

All three vaccines confer comparable protection against the disease so the only differences between them are the routes of administration, dose schedules and adverse effects.

It is therefore reasonable to advise the following:

● Individuals who have had the whole-cell vaccine in the past could continue having the same vaccine for their boosters but perhaps ID.

● If the patient prefers the oral route for vaccination, or if there is a need to minimize side effects, the oral typhoid vaccine can be used.

● When the primary course is to be given parenterally, the typhim Vi vaccine is preferable as it involves only a single injection.

Typhoid infection

This is a potentially lethal infection that follows ingestion of *Salmonella typhi*. The incubation period is 1–3 weeks. It can affect any age but usually it occurs in older children and adults. The onset is insidious with headaches and lethargy being the usual presenting symptoms. It then progresses to myalgia, abdominal discomfort, cough, malaise, constipation and later bloody diarrhoea with rigors. A characteristic rash ('rose spots') may appear.

About 2% of patients will continue harbouring the organism in their gallbladder after infection for many years, becoming chronic carriers and excreting it periodically in their stools.

Typhoid fever is acquired through contaminated food and drink. Spread is usually faecal–oral. Food and water can be contaminated by excreta of a human case of typhoid or a chronic carrier. Sewage and water supplies can be important sources of infection. It is, therefore, predominantly a disease of countries economically underdeveloped, with poor sanitation, while it is uncommon in the affluent parts of the world.

Eradication of typhoid in the community involves the provision of pure clean water, proper sewage disposal systems, identification and treatment of chronic carriers and immunization.

Approximately 200 cases of typhoid are reported each year in the UK, most of them travellers returning from abroad, especially the Indian subcontinent. Some cases are contracted in the UK from carriers who were exposed to the disease abroad.

Typhoid vaccination is recommended for travel to all countries except northern and western Europe, North America, Japan, Australia and New Zealand. It is also recommended for laboratory workers handling specimens which may contain typhoid organisms.

Cholera

Contraindications to vaccination
● Acute febrile illness.
● Chronic illness — patients in remission may relapse as a result of an adverse reaction to vaccination with whole-cell vaccine.
● Severe reaction to a previously administered dose of the vaccine.
● Children under the age of 1 year — reactions are more frequent in this age group.
● Pregnancy is a relative contraindication and the vaccine may be given if there is a clear risk of infection.
● Yellow fever vaccination should be separated from cholera vaccination by at least 3 weeks, or if not, they should be given simultaneously (possible inhibition of antibody response to both vaccines).

Possible side and adverse effects

Local reactions
Transient redness, swelling, pain and induration lasting from 1 to 2 days.

General reactions
Headaches, pyrexia and malaise usually lasting for 24–48 h. Anaphylactic reaction and neurological symptoms such as neuritis, polyneuritis, cerebral and meningeal irritation may occur very rarely.

The vaccine
It contains heat-killed phenol-preserved *Vibrio cholerae*, serotypes Inaba and Ogawa, at a concentration of 8 000 000 000 organisms per millilitre. It protects against both the classical and El Tor biotypes. On standing, the preparation has a tendency to settle out in a gelatinous form. Vigorous shaking is necessary to resuspend the vaccine.

Administration
● The first dose of the primary course is given by deep SC or IM injection, while the second dose and subsequent boosters may be given ID in order to minimize systemic reaction.

Table 43 Administration specifications for cholera vaccine

Age	Primary course			Second dose and boosters		Booster interval
	First dose IM/SC (ml)	Time interval		IM/SC (ml)	ID (ml)	
1–5 years	0.1			0.3	0.1	
5–10 years	0.3	4 weeks (minimum 1 week)		0.5	0.1	6 months
Over 10 years and adults	0.5			1	0.2	

● The primary course consists of two doses 4 weeks apart (minimum 1 week).

● Immunity is short-lived and the vaccine should be given every 6 months as long as the subject is likely to be exposed to infection. A single booster dose will suffice even if longer than 6 months has elapsed.

● Repeated vaccination over a period of a few years may result in the development of hypersensitivity to protein constituents of the vaccine.

● The vaccine protects 50% of vaccinees for 3–6 months.

● Although cholera vaccination is not required for international travel, travellers to or from certain countries which have reported cholera infection may be required by border officials acting unofficially to produce evidence of recent cholera vaccination. Travellers who lack such written evidence risk having to receive the vaccine at the border, sometimes with needles of questionable sterility.

● A Cholera International Certificate is valid for 6 months after the first dose of the primary course (some countries may insist on two doses and/or non-ID administration) and immediately after a booster dose.

● The risk areas are Central and South America, Africa, the Middle East and Asia.

Vaccine availability
Cholera Vaccine BP, Evans Medical Ltd, available in multidose vials of 1.5 and 10 ml — discard partly used vaccine vials.

Storage: Between +2 and +8°C. *Do not freeze.* Protect from light.

Cholera infection
This is caused by the enterotoxin producing *Vibrio cholerae*, a Gram-

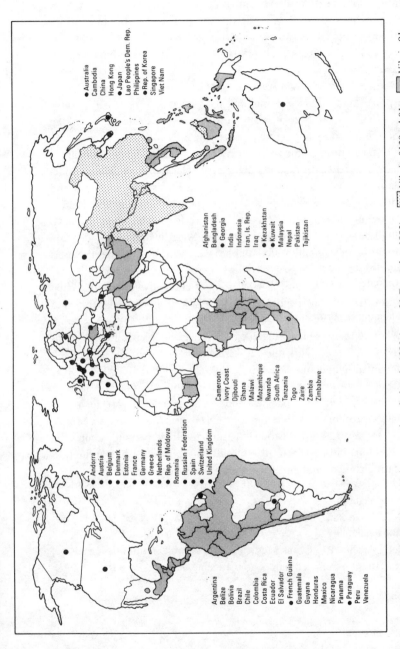

Fig. 9 Countries, or areas within countries, reporting cholera in 1993 (as at 31 December 1993). ░ Vibrio 0139 ad 01; ▓ Vibrio 01; ● imported cases only. Reproduced with permission from the WHO.

Australia
Cambodia
China
Hong Kong
Japan
Lao People's Dem. Rep.
Philippines
Rep. of Korea
Singapore
Viet Nam

Afghanistan
Bangladesh
Georgia
India
Indonesia
Iran, Is. Rep.
Iraq
Kazakhstan
Kuwait
Malaysia
Nepal
Pakistan
Tajikistan

Cameroon
Ivory Coast
Djibouti
Ghana
Malawi
Mozambique
Rwanda
South Africa
Tanzania
Togo
Zaire
Zambia
Zimbabwe

Andorra
Austria
Belgium
Denmark
Estonia
France
Germany
Greece
Netherlands
Rep. of Moldova
Romania
Russian Federation
Spain
Switzerland
United Kingdom

Argentina
Belize
Bolivia
Brazil
Chile
Colombia
Costa Rica
Ecuador
El Salvador
French Guiana
Guatemala
Guyana
Honduras
Mexico
Nicaragua
Panama
Paraguay
Peru
Venezuela

negative, comma-shaped rod that has two biotypes: the El Tor (now predominant) and the classical (it can still be found in the Indian sub-continent where it has caused numerous epidemics during the past 200 years). Inaba and Ogawa are serotypes based on O (or somatic) anti-genic determinants.

Cholera is predominantly a disease of countries with poor sanitation and poor standards of personal and food hygiene (Fig. 9). It is trans-mitted by ingestion of contaminated water or food. Adequate cooking of food and boiling of water eradicates the organism.

The incubation period ranges from a few hours to 5 days. The illness is characterized by the sudden onset of painless, profuse, watery diar-rhoea that leads to dehydration, metabolic acidosis, hypokalaemia and hypovolaemic shock. Mild or asymptomatic infection can also occur.

In recent epidemics in Latin America, raw fish and seafood products, vegetables that had been irrigated with raw waste water, and inadequate chlorination of drinking water supplies were identified as main sources and causes.

In 1991 and 1992, over 500 000 cases of cholera were reported each year to WHO, of which approximately 70% occur in Latin America and nearly 30% in Africa.

About 60 cases of cholera have been reported in England and Wales during the past 12 years and all were contracted overseas — the last documented indigenous case was in 1893.

Cholera is undoubtedly a disease of poverty and the risk to travellers, especially on a package holiday, is very small. WHO no longer recommends cholera vaccination for travel to and from cholera endemic areas. However, border officials acting unofficially (and sometimes officially) may insit on a valid International Certificate of Vaccination indicating cholera immunization within 6 months.

Rabies

Contraindications to vaccination
- Acute febrile illness.
- Severe general reaction to a previously administered rabies vaccine.
- Severe sensitivity to neomycin or β-propiolactone.
- Pregnancy, unless there is a significant risk of infection in which case the importance of the vaccination may outweigh the possible risk to the fetus.

Possible side and adverse effects

Local reaction
Swelling, redness and pain may develop within 24–48 h from administration.

General reactions
Myalgia, headaches, fever, vomiting or urticarial rash within 24 h from administration. Very rarely Guillain–Barré syndrome and anaphylactic shock.

The vaccine
Viral vaccine inactivated by β-propiolactone vaccine. It is a freeze-dried suspension of Wistar rabies virus strain, cultured on human diploid cells.

Administration
The dose is the same for all ages. It should be given by IM or deep SC injection. It is free in the UK (on the NHS) for people at occupational risk (see below), though it is not available on the NHS for routine immunization of travellers, who should be issued with a private prescription.
- The three-dose course brings the UK into line with other European countries. For those people going on a one-off trip, the old two-dose regime (0 and 28 days) may give adequate protection.
- The three-dose course causes seroconversion virtually in all recipients. It is, therefore, unnecessary to test seroconversion routinely,

Table 44 Pre-exposure immunization for rabies

Immunization	Dose (ml)	Route	Schedule (days)
First dose	1		0
Second dose	1	IM or SC	7
Third dose	1		28
Booster	1		Every 2–3 years

except in travellers taking chloroquine antimalarial prophylaxis, in whom the immune response may be hampered. On the other hand individuals exposed to the virus should have regular 6-monthly antibody testing.

● The painful abdominal injections were abandoned in the mid-1970s. The new human diploid cell vaccine is almost painless. It should be administered into the deltoid region (avoid the gluteal region) and in children in the anterolateral aspect of the thigh.

● The vaccine is available free on the NHS for the following people at occupational risk (as suggested by the DoH in its publication, *Immunization against Infectious Disease*, HMSO, 1992):

    (a) at animal quarantine centres;

    (b) at zoos;

    (c) at research and acclimatization centres where primates and other imported animals are housed;

    (d) at ports, e.g. Custom and Excise officers;

    (e) agents authorized to carry imported animals;

    (f) veterinary and technical staff at government offices (agriculture, food and fisheries);

    (g) local authority inspectors appointed under the Diseases of Animals Act;

    (h) veterinary staff and zoologists working abroad; and

    (i) health workers who may come into close contact with a patient with rabies.

● The first dose of the vaccine should be given as soon as possible after the suspected contact (day 0). Human rabies immunoglobulin is only necessary if the person with the suspected contact has not previously been fully immunized.

● Immediately after exposure wash lesions copiously and thoroughly with soap and running water for at least 5 min. Do not suture wound

Table 45 Post-exposure treatment for rabies

Immunization status	Dose (ml)	Route	Schedule (days)	Rabies-specific immunoglobulin 20 IU/kg bodyweight
Fully immunized	1	IM or SC	0, 3 to 7 (two doses)	Unnecessary
Unimmunized	1	IM or SC	0, 3, 7, 14, 30, 90 (six doses)	Half infiltrated around the wound, the rest IM

immediately. Local medical advice should be sought regarding vaccination.

● In the case of domestic animals, advise the patient to ask to see the last vaccination certificate. The animal should be observed for 10 days. Exchange addresses/telephone numbers so that the casualty can be notified should the animal begin to behave abnormally. Inform the local police and own GP on return.

● If the animal is wild or stray, inform the local police. The local doctor will advise whether post-exposure treatment is necessary.

Vaccine availability

● Rabies Vaccine BP, Pasteur, Merieux UK Ltd, available in single-dose vial with disposable syringe containing 1 ml of diluent.

The Public Health Laboratory Services (Virus Reference Division) or the Communicable Disease Surveillance Centres will supply the free vaccine for those at occupational risk.

Storage: Between +2 and +8°C. *Do not freeze.*

Rabies infection

Rabies is an acute encephalomyelitic virus infection, that produces an acute febrile illness with rapidly progressive central nervous system symptoms. There can be hydrophobia, dysphagia, hallucinations, convulsions, paralysis and almost always (untreated) ends in death.

The virus is transmitted to humans by the bite of an infected animal, rarely through mucous membranes. Most animals when infected, become ill within 3 days hence the 10-day standard period of observation of a suspected animal. Other modes of transmission are by transplantation, e.g. corneas, or air-borne (migrating bats).

In Europe the red fox is predominantly infected, except in Turkey where dogs make up the most registered cases (and human cases are relatively more common). Apart from foxes and dogs, other animals that can become infected are cats, bats, deer, badgers, horses, cattle, skunks, raccoons and others.

The incubation period in humans ranges from 5 days to over 1 year (average 2 months).

Rabies can be found in most countries except the UK, Eire, Scandinavia, some Caribbean and Polynesian countries, Australia and New Zealand.

The last indigenous case in the UK was in 1902, and all subsequent non-indigenous cases have been imported. Between 1977 and 1987 six cases were reported in the UK, three of them in children bitten by dogs on the Indian subcontinent. In contrast, in 1992, 12 cases of human rabies were reported in Europe (11 in the former Soviet Union and one in France — imported from Algeria). During the same year the animal rabies cases reported in Europe were 11 000 (66% in foxes).

The current strategy for the elimination of rabies in Europe is by vaccinating domestic animals parenterally and by oral vaccination of foxes. Distribution of attenuated live vaccine is via impregnated chicken heads acting as bait. A new bait consisting of fat and fish meal has improved the seroconversion rate and facilitated mass production.

Countries free of rabies impose strict control in animal traffic across borders. Animals that are brought in legally are isolated and placed under observation — for 6 months in the UK.

Meningococcus A and C

Contraindications to vaccination
● Acute febrile illness.
● Severe reaction to a previously administered dose of the vaccine.
● Children under the age of 2 months as they do not generally respond to the vaccine.
● Pregnancy, unless there is a significant risk of infection, in which case the importance of vaccination may outweigh the possible risk to the fetus.

Possible side and adverse effects

Local reactions
Swelling, redness and pain, lasting for 1–2 days.

General reactions
Irritability, fever and rigors in the first 24–48 h. Anaphylaxis is very rare.

The vaccine
An inactivated polysaccharide vaccine against *Neisseria meningitidis* serogroups A and C. Each 0.5 ml dose of reconstituted vaccine contains 50 μg of each purified bacterial capsular polysaccharide.

Administration
● Neither of the two vaccines available are effective against meningococcus group B, the strain most commonly found in the UK.
● After a single injection, the earliest protective antibodies can appear is 5–7 days (important when travelling or attempting to control an epidemic (see seroconversion in Tables 46 and 47).
● The vaccine may not induce an effective response in the immunosuppressed.
● Children under 18 months of age show poor response to the vaccine. In case of travel to areas where the risk of meningococcal meningitis A or C is high, such children should be vaccinated but another dose of the

Table 46 A C V A X (SmithKline Beecham)

Age	Dose (ml)	Route	Seroconversion (older children/ adults)	Immunity	
				>5 years old	<5 years old
Adults and children from 2 months	0.5	Deep SC	>90% within 14–21 days	5 years	1–2 years

Table 47 Meningivac A + C (Merieux)

Age	Dose (ml)	Route	Seroconversion	Immunity
Adults and children from 18 months	0.5	Deep SC or IM	>90% within 5–14 days	3 years

vaccine should be given at the age of 18 months or 3 months afterwards, whichever is first (Meningivac A + C) or 1–2 years afterwards (A C V A X).

● The vaccines are available on N H S prescription.

Indications

● *Post-splenectomy* and especially before the operation if it is an elective procedure.

● *Close contacts* of cases of meningococcal meningitis caused by group A or C should be given the vaccine in addition to chemoprophylaxis. It is ineffective in cases where the group B organism has caused the disease.

● *In outbreaks* of meningococcal disease caused by group A and/or C in schools, playgroups, etc., immunization of contacts should be considered.

● *Travellers* to endemic areas are recommended vaccination. These areas are mainly countries in the 'meningitis belt' of Africa, running from Kenya in the east, to Senegal in the west: Kenya, Uganda, Central African Republic, Cameroon, Nigeria, Ivory Coast, Liberia, northern parts of Sierra Leone, Gambia, Guinea, Togo, Benin, southern Senegal, Mali, Niger, Chad, Sudan and south-west Ethiopia (Fig. 10).

● In addition to the above countries recommended by the international division of the DoH, W H O is also advising immunization for travellers to Burundi, Tanzania and Zambia, reflecting a southwards extension of the high-risk areas.

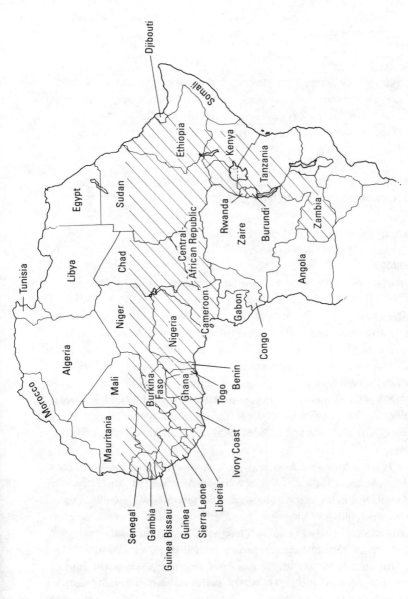

Fig. 10 'Meningitis belt' of Africa with recent extension to Burundi, Tanzania and Zambia.

• Travellers to Mecca, Saudi Arabia during the Haj are recommended vaccination and certification — the certificate of vaccination needs to be issued not more than 3 years, and not less than 10 days, before arrival in Saudi Arabia. Sporadic outbreaks of group A disease also occur in India, Nepal and Brazil.

Vaccine availability

• AC VAX, SmithKline Beecham Pharmaceuticals, available as monodose vials and 10-dose vials, each with separate ampoule/vial of diluent. After reconstitution, use within 4 h.

• Meningivac A + C, Merieux UK Ltd, available as a single-dose vial of vaccine with a syringe of diluent (0.5 ml). After reconstitution, use within 1 h. Shake before use.

Vaccines are available from the Public Health Laboratory Services (PHLS) Meningococcal Reference Laboratory.

Storage. Between +2 and + 8°C. *Do not freeze diluent.*

Meningococcal infections

Neisseria meningitidis, the causative organism, is a Gram-negative diplococcus with 12 serogroups identified as A, B, C, X, Y, Z, W135, 29E, H, I, K and L. The relative importance of the causative serogroups also varies with age, 70% of cases under 5 years are attributable to group B in the UK, but this falls to 50% in those over 10 years of age (J.K. Williams & J. Burnie (1987) *Bacterial Meningitis*, pp. 93–115. Academic Press).

Of all (1398) isolates submitted to the British PHLS Meningococcal Reference Laboratory in 1991, group B strains accounted for 69%, group C for 28% and group A for 0.4% (*PHLS Communicable Disease Report* 1992; 2 (6)).

Frequent epidemics associated with group A occur in the 'meningitis belt' of Africa, India, Brazil and Saudi Arabia. The outbreaks are generally in the hot dry season, therefore, in Africa they occur mainly in the first 4 months of the year.

Infection is acquired by inhaling infected droplets of respiratory secretions or by direct contact with a patient or carrier. About one in four young adults may be carriers while the rate in the general population is one in 10. The incubation period is from 1–10 days, most commonly less than 4 days.

Humans are the only known carrier of the meningococcus (in the upper respiratory tract) and act as a reservoir for transmission of the disease.

Meningococcal infections occur most frequently in children younger than 5 years with peak incidence at 6–12 months. Headaches, nausea, vomiting, fever, photophobia, stiff neck and a petechial or purpuric rash are the classical signs of meningococcal disease. The onset can be insidious or fulminant as in the case of septicaemia. The mortality rate is about 3–5% for those with meningitis and 15–20% for those with meningococcal septicaemia. Close contacts of patients with meningococcal disease are at increased risk of developing infection.

Prevention

A patient with meningococcal disease should be isolated. The main preventive measures are chemoprophylaxis administered to close contacts and immunization if serogroups A or C are suspected. The vaccine has no effect on group B. Hopes of control of serogroup B meningococci by immunization are rising with attempts to develop a vaccine. Such a vaccine was developed from a Cuban epidemic strain of the organism (in 1992). The results from the use of this vaccine were encouraging but its usefulness in preventing epidemic serogroup B meningococcal disease was questionable (*Lancet* 1992; 340; 1074–8). The existing vaccine (A and C strains) is least protective for those at greatest risk (under 2-year-old children) and does not prevent nasal carriage.

At present most authorities do not recommend routine immunization with the existing vaccine of serogroups A and C. On the other hand, close contacts of cases of meningococcal meningitis A or C should be considered for immunization in addition to appropriate chemoprophylaxis.

Notes

Tick-borne encephalitis

Contraindications to vaccination
- Acute febrile illness.
- Severe sensitivity (anaphylactic reaction) to the preservative thiomersal or to egg protein.
- Severe hypersensitivity to a previously administered tick-borne encephalitis vaccine.

Possible side and adverse effects

Local reactions
Swelling, redness and pain around the injection site and swelling of the regional lymphatic glands.

General reactions
Pyrexia may occur, especially in children, not usually over 38°C and lasting up to 24 h following mainly the first dose of the vaccine. Rarely neuritis.

The vaccine
Viral inactivated vaccine. It is not licensed in the UK, therefore available on a 'named patient' basis only.

Administration
- There is no age limit for vaccination but babies should only be vaccinated if there is actual risk of infection. The dose is the same for all ages and the primary course consists of three doses of the vaccine.

Table 49 Administration specifications for tick-borne encephalitis vaccine

Immunization	Dose (ml)	Route	Schedule (months)
First dose	0.5	IM	0
Second dose	0.5	IM	1–3
Third dose	0.5	IM	9–12
Booster	0.5	IM	Every 3 years

● In vaccinees up to the age of 30, seroconversion may reach 100%, and in the over-60s, seroconversion of 93% can be achieved after the third dose.

● Immunization should preferably be given in the winter months. If it is started in late spring or early summer (during seasonal tick activity), it is recommended that the second dose is given 2 weeks after the first, in order to seroconvert as soon as possible.

● The vaccine is not contraindicated in pregnant women.

● Immunosuppressed patients should have their antibody titre checked 4 weeks after the second dose of the vaccine. Repeat the second dose if at this stage seroconversion is unsatisfactory.

Vaccine availability

FSME–IMMUN Inject Vaccine, Immuno Ltd, available in prefilled syringe containing 0.5 ml suspension. Available on a 'named patient' basis. Shelf life of 1 year.

Storage: Between +2 and +8°C. *Do not freeze.*

Tick-borne encephalitis immunoglobulin

Tick-borne encephalitis-specific immunoglobulin is available for post-exposure prophylaxis of unimmunized (whether by choice, where the vaccine is contraindicated or the first injection was given 1–4 days before infection) and immunosuppressed persons. It can be administered before exposure and up to 96 h after exposure, i.e. after a tick bite in a tick-borne encephalitis endemic area.

Immunoglobulin availability

FSME-Bulin specific immunoglobulin, Immuno Ltd, available in vials containing 1, 2, 5 or 10 ml.

Storage: Between +2 and +8°C.

Tick-borne encephalitis infection

Tick-borne encephalitis is one of the arbovirus infections (others are yellow fever and Japanese B encephalitis). It is transmitted by the bite of infected *Ixodes* ticks which feed on a wide range of birds and forest mammals. The incubation is about 10 days, and the effects vary from subclinical infection through a febrile illness to frank encephalitis. Recovery without sequelae is the general rule.

Its distribution is mainly in low warm forested areas, especially with heavy undergrowth, in parts of former Yugoslavia, Czech and Slovak Republics, Germany, Austria, Poland, Scandinavia and the Commonwealth of Independent States (the former Soviet Union).

The travellers who might be particularly at risk are campers and walkers in Alpine meadowland, in late spring and early summer.

Prevention is by avoiding tick bites (insect repellents can be of some use) and by immunization with tick-borne encephalitis vaccine.

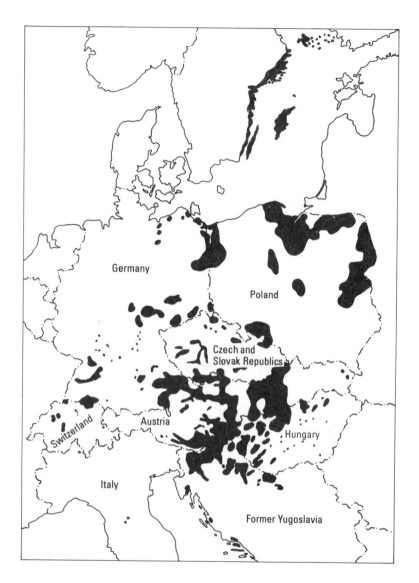

Fig. 11 Distribution of tick-borne encephalitis. ▆ .

Japanese B encephalitis

Contraindications to vaccination
- Acute febrile illness.
- Severe sensitivity to a previously administered Japanese B encephalitis vaccine.
- Cardiac, hepatic and renal conditions, especially during acute exacerbations.
- Diabetes.
- Immunodeficiency and malignancy.
- Pregnancy, unless the pregnant woman is travelling to an endemic area of very high risk of infection.

Possible side and adverse effects

Local reactions
Swelling, redness and pain.

General reactions
Headaches, rigors, fever, rarely urticaria and angioneurotic oedema.

The vaccine
Viral inactivated vaccine derived from mouse brain, on a named patient basis (not licensed in the U K).

Administration
- The two doses of the primary course can be given 1–2 weeks apart

Table 49 Administration specifications for Japanese B encephalitis vaccine

Age	Dose (ml)	Route	Schedule (days)	Booster
Children under 3 years	0.5	SC	0, 7, 28	1–4 years
Adults and children over 3 years	1	SC	0, 7, 28	1–4 years

and give protection for up to 3 months. The third dose (at 28 days) is especially recommended for the over 60s because of their relatively lower antibody response to the vaccination, and for those intending to visit highly endemic areas.

● It may take up to 1 month after the primary course for immunity to develop.

Vaccine availability
Lyophilized Japanese B Encephalitis Vaccine Biken, Cambridge Self-care Diagnostics Ltd, available in single-dose vials for reconstitution. Available on a named patient basis.

Storage: Below 10°C. *Do not freeze.*

Japanese B encephalitis infection
It is an uncommon but serious arboviral infection that is endemic throughout most of the Far East and South-East Asia.

The hosts are mainly pigs, migrating birds and ducks. Transmission to humans is by bite of infected rice field breeding mosquitoes of the genus *Culex*. One in 200 infections becomes clinically apparent and the case fatality rate in epidemics is estimated at 10–50%, with about half the survivors being left with neurological damage. The peak season is the summer monsoon months (June–September).

Prevention is by avoiding mosquito bites and by immunization. Vaccination is recommended for travellers to endemic areas of South-East Asia and the Far East if one of the following conditions applies:

● visit during the summer monsoon months;

● visitors to rural areas whatever the length of their visit;

● visitors staying more than 1 month irrespective of rural or urban abode; or

● frequent visitors (e.g. those engaged in trade or commerce) to cities surrounded by endemic areas.

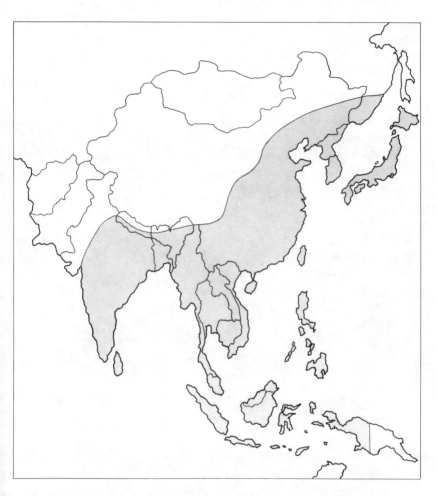

Fig. 12 Endemicity of Japanese B encephalitis in South-East Asia, ☐.

Notes

Varicella

Human varicella-zoster immunoglobulin

Contraindications to immunoglobulin
- In patients with thrombocytopenia.
- It must not be given IV.
- Severe hypersensitivity to thiomersal.
- Previous anaphylactic reaction following administration of human varicella–zoster immunoglobulin.

Possible side and adverse effects

Local reactions. Short-term discomfort at the site of injection.

General reactions. Very rarely anaphylaxis especially in patients who have had an atypical reaction to blood transfusion or treatment with plasma derivatives, and in patients who have antibodies to IgA.

The immunoglobulin
Human varicella–zoster immunoglobulin (HVZIG) is manufactured from pooled plasma of blood donors with high titres of varicella zoster antibody.

Each plasma donation and the final product are tested by validated procedures and found non-reactive for hepatitis B surface antigen and also antibodies to HIV-1.

Administration
- It is available in a single-dose vial of 250 mg for strictly IM use.
- Human varicella-zoster immunoglobulin does not prevent infection if given within 72 h of exposure, but may attenuate an attack if given within 10 days after exposure.
- Of all adults in the UK over the age of 20, 95% show evidence of previous infection with varicella zoster virus (VZV). Contacts of immunosuppressed patients without a definite history of chickenpox should be screened for antibody to the virus.

Table 50 Human varicella-zoster immunoglobulin dosage

Age	Dose (mg)	Route
0–5 years	250	IM
6–10 years	500	IM
11–14 years	750	IM
> 15 years and adults	1000	IM

- The DoH in its book *Immunization against Infectious Disease* (HMSO, 1992) recommends human varicella-zoster immunoglobulin for individuals in contact with chicken pox or shingles in the following groups:

    (a) immunocompromised patients by disease or treatment who are seronegative for VZV antibody;

    (b) bone marrow transplant recipients regardless of history of chickenpox;

    (c) symptomatic HIV positive individuals unless known to have VZV antibodies (asymptomatic HIV positive individuals in contact with chickenpox or shingles do not require the immunoglobulin);

    (d) patients with debilitating disease;

    (e) infants up to 4 weeks after birth whose mothers develop chickenpox (not shingles) in the period 7 days before to 1 month after delivery;

    (f) infants in contact with chickenpox or shingles whose mothers have no history of chickenpox or who on testing have no antibody;

    (g) premature infants in contact with chickenpox or shingles, born before 30 weeks of gestation or with a birthweight of less than 1 kg — even if the mother gives a positive history of chickenpox they may not possess maternal antibody; or

    (h) pregnant women without a history of chickenpox who are found not to possess antibody to the virus. About two-thirds of pregnant women have antibody despite a negative history. This immunoglobulin does not prevent infection but it may attenuate maternal disease.

- The following infants, aged less than 1 month, will possess antibody to the virus, therefore they do *not* require the immunoglobulin:

    (a) born more than 7 days after the onset of maternal chickenpox;

    (b) whose mothers have a positive history of chickenpox and/or a positive antibody result (with the exception of premature infants as described above); or

(c) whose mothers develop zoster before or after delivery.

● Particular attention should be paid to patients receiving high doses of corticosteroids (child on 2 or more mg/kg per day of prednisolone, adult on over 60 mg/day). Do not stop the corticosteroid. Administer the immunoglobulin (unless shown to have antibody to the virus) and seek prompt specialist care and urgent treatment (e.g. systemic acyclovir).

Immunoglobulin availability

● Human Varicella-Zoster Immunoglobulin (IM), Bio Products Laboratory, available in 250 mg single-dose vial. For NHS use only it can be obtained from all public health laboratory services or from The Laboratories, Belfast City Hospital.

Storage: Between +2 and +8°C. *Do not freeze.*

Varicella vaccine

An unlicensed live attenuated varicella vaccine is available from SmithKline Beecham on a 'named patient' basis, for immunocompromised patients such as children with leukaemia, about to have kidney transplants, etc.

The Oka strain of live attenuated varicella vaccine was developed in the early 1970s in Japan for use in immunocompromised children at risk of varicella.

Two doses of the vaccine, 3 months apart, are given to immunocompromised patients. Maintenance chemotherapy is withheld for 1 week before and 1 week after the first dose of the vaccine, while steroids are withheld for an additional week. Efficacy of the vaccine is estimated at 85%.

About 90% of healthy children are protected after one dose of the vaccine (a suggestion is to incorporate varicella immunization at 15 months of age for all children), while in healthy young adults, protection is about 70% after two doses. A vaccinee who is not completely protected from chickenpox usually has a modified illness after exposure to infection.

Vaccine-induced immunity is estimated at 6–10 years. About 25% of adults and immunocompromised children and adults will lose detectable antibodies within 1 year from vaccination. It is of concern that these individuals might then become exposed to wild-type virus and get severe varicella.

The Japanese have licensed varicella vaccine for use in healthy children. In the UK, the vaccine is still unlicensed.

Varicella and zoster infection

Varicella (chickenpox) is a highly infectious disease with humans being the only reservoir of the virus. It is caused by the herpesvirus varicella zoster virus and primary infection results in chickenpox. The virus persists in a latent form and reactivation results in herpes zoster (shingles).

The virus is transmitted directly by personal contact with chickenpox or shingles lesions or by air-borne droplet infection. Most cases of chickenpox occur in children between 5 and 10 years. In children it is usually a mild disease, much less severe than in adults. The infection can be severe in immunocompromised patients, in neonates and in pregnant women particularly in the first trimester (fetal varicella syndrome).

Virtually everyone in the UK has had the infection by the age of 40 years. Most adults (up to 95%) with negative or unknown history of chickenpox are likely to be immune.

The incubation period is usually 2–3 weeks. Patients are contagious 1–2 days before the characteristic vesicles appear and until they dry.

The complications of primary varicella disease include pneumonitis, haemorrhagic problems, meningoencephalitis, pyogenic sepsis, fetal varicella syndrome when infection occurs in the first trimester (microcephaly, cataracts, limb hypoplasia, growth retardation). Reactivated varicella (shingles) can cause blindness, post-herpetic neuralgia and encephalitis (approximately one in five people develop shingles at some time in their lives).

Chickenpox in children does not require specific treatment unless severe and in immunocompromised patients who should receive human varicella-zoster immunoglobulin IM and oral acyclovir (20 mg/kg bodyweight, to a maximum of 800 mg, started within 24 h of onset of rash and repeated at 6-hourly intervals for 5 days). If a patient is on corticosteroids, they should not be stopped — seek specialist advice. Adults with severe chickenpox or shingles could also receive acyclovir. Famciclovir is licensed also for the treatment of herpes zoster in adults. For indications of varicella-zoster immunoglobulin, see p. 150.

The latest UK figures show that chickenpox causes nearly 30 deaths a year, and one-third of these are associated with immunosuppression.

Plague

Contraindications to vaccination
- Acute febrile illness.
- Severe reaction to a previously administered dose of the vaccine.
- Severe hypersensitivity (anaphylactic reaction) to phenol, beef protein and soya casein.

Possible side and adverse effects

Local reactions
Swelling, redness and pain in approximately 10% of vaccinees.

General reactions
Headaches, fever, malaise and lymphadenopathy. Rarely urticaria and sterile abscesses.

The vaccine
Formaline-inactivated whole-cell *Yersinia pestis* vaccine, has been grown in artificial media and preserved in phenol.

Administration
- The vaccine is administered by deep SC or IM injection.
- Seroconversion is estimated at 92%.
- Recommended for:
   (a) laboratory workers, geologists or biologists working directly with *Yersinia pestis* infected animals;

Table 51 Immunization with plague vaccine

First dose	Second dose	Third dose	Immediate boosters	Further boosters
1 ml	0.2 ml 1 month after first	0.2 ml 3 months after first	Three booster doses 0.2 ml each, every 6 months	0.2 ml every 1–2 years

(b) long stay travellers to endemic areas where the risk of contracting the disease is high;

(c) workers travelling to disaster endemic areas; or

(d) soldiers in endemic areas.

- It is not recommended for routine immunization of travellers.

Vaccine availability

The vaccine is not available in the UK and has to be imported from the USA for a 'named patient' basis only. Contact Geer Laboratories Inc (see p. 216). Readers in the UK should note that Bayer PLC are no longer able to supply the vaccine.

Plague infection

The name plague is derived from the Greek *plaga/plege* which means a 'blow' or 'wound'. It is known in the West as the Black Death.

It is caused by *Yersinia pestis*, a bipolar strain, Gram-negative rod. It infects rodents and other animals. About 30 different kinds of fleas can transport the bacterium from one animal host to another (humans are a host too).

Bubonic plague is transmitted by the bite of an infected flea or rodent while pneumonic plague is transmitted by aerosols during direct contact with an infected patient or an infected animal.

The incubation time is 2–6 days for the bubonic plague and slightly shorter for the pneumonic variety. Symptoms include fever, headaches, myalgia, rigors and pain in the groin because of the lymphadenopathy. The condition can progress to septicaemia. The onset of symptoms is usually sudden, appearing 2–7 days after the flea bite. The organism can be isolated in blood cultures, cerebrospinal fluid or in sputum. It is sensitive to tetracycline and streptomycin.

Plague can be found in the western USA, parts of South America, Asia and Africa. In Zaire there have been new reports recently of hundreds of cases of bubonic plague and over 200 deaths.

In 1990 there were 7631 cases reported in 19 countries and 570 deaths. Among countries reporting cases are the US (10–30 cases/year), Kenya, Equador and Peru.

Control of fleas and suppression of the rodent population are important epidemic measures in countries which face the problem of plague.

Malaria

Malaria is one of the more common and serious of the tropical diseases. Almost half of the world's population is at risk. There are probably up to 100 000 000 clinical cases of malaria and over 1 000 000 deaths every year, the majority of them in Africa.

About 1600–2000 cases of malaria are 'imported' into the UK each year with *Plasmodium falciparum* malaria cases steadily rising. There were 12 deaths in 1991 and 10 in 1992 from malaria in the UK.

Epidemiology

Malaria in humans is caused by one of four *Plasmodium* species (mean incubation period): *P. falciparum* (12 days), *P. vivax* (13 days), *P. ovale* (17 days) and *P. malariae* (28 days).

Infection is usually acquired by the bite of an infected female *Anopheles* mosquito. Other less common modes of transmission include blood transfusion, contaminated needles and congenital infection.

Unless properly treated *Plasmodium* persists in a dormant stage causing periodic relapses for as long as 1 year (*P. falciparum*), 4 years (*P. vivax* and *P. ovale*) and even over 30 years (*P. malariae*). It is important, therefore, to recognize that malarial illness may be delayed until several weeks or months after exposure. Equally important to remember is the fact that the minimum incubation period of malaria is about 12 days so holiday-makers are most likely to develop the disease after their return.

Frequent travel to endemic areas does not convey useful immunity against malaria. Only those people who have survived childhood in a malaria-endemic area may be considered to be immune as long as they do not leave that area for more than a few months. Immigrants resident for some years in the UK who then visit their home country can be susceptible to severe malaria.

P. falciparum is developing resistance to antimalarial drugs and the mosquito host is becoming resistant to insecticides, enjoying an increase in breeding sites due to deforestation and irrigation projects.

Clinical presentation

The classic symptoms are malaise, myagia, headaches, high fever, rigors and sweats. Other symptoms can be nausea, vomiting, diarrhoea, abdominal pain, back pain, arthralgia and jaundice caused by haemolysis and anaemia. Severe infections can result in severe anaemia, renal and hepatic failure, coagulopathy, convulsions, encephalopathy, coma and death. Fever fluctuates so a patient may be afebrile when seen.

Pregnant women should be discouraged from travelling to endemic areas as the infection in pregnancy poses serious problems such as miscarriage, stillbirth and risk of maternal death.

Diagnosis

By microscopic examination of stained fresh blood film. Negative findings do not exclude malaria entirely and further samples should be examined in the presence of clinical suspicion. Serological tests for antibodies against individual *Plasmodium* species cannot differentiate current from past infection, therefore, these tests are of limited use in the diagnosis of acute malaria.

Treatment

The GP should consider admission to hospital of cases where malaria is suspected or proven, especially *P. falciparum* malaria because of the risk of complications.

Here are three possible regimens of oral antimalarial drugs:

● Quinine sulphate (300 mg tablet) 600 mg three times daily for adults (10 mg/kg bodyweight three times daily for children) for 7 days, during which a single dose is given of sulfadoxine/pyrimethamine (Fansidar) — three tablets for adults (children: up to 4 years, half a tablet; 5–6 years, one tablet; 7–9 years, one and a half tablets; 10–14 years, two tablets); avoid if patient is allergic to sulphonamide. If there has been previous sensitivity to Fansidar, use doxycycline 200 mg once, then 100 mg daily for 6 days (not for a child under 12 years or for a pregnant woman).

● Mefloquine (Lariam 250 mg tablet) 20 mg of base/kg (maximum: 1500 mg) divided into two doses 6–8 h apart (not for pregnant women, patients with psychiatric disease or epilepsy, or on β-blockers, digoxin, calcium channel blockers, quinidine or metoclopramide).

● Halofantrine (Halfan 250 mg tablet) 500 mg for adults, 8 mg/kg for children, every 6 h for three doses; repeat after 1 week.

Prophylaxis

Immunization

The development of the ideal malaria vaccine is beset by the complexities of the different stages in the life cycle of the malaria parasite and the differing needs and responses to a vaccine in different populations.

The best and most promising results of a vaccine to date have been obtained by the Bogota, Colombia group (*Lancet* 1993; 341: 705–10). In a randomized blind trial, a synthetic vaccine protected a group of children against malaria. It is to be hoped that this initial promise will be sustained.

General advice to travellers

● Take chemoprophylaxis against malaria, starting 1 week before arrival and continuing without interruption until at least 4 weeks after leaving the malarious area.

● Comply with chemoprophylaxis; nearly three-quarters of travellers who develop malaria do so because they do not comply or do not take chemoprophylaxis. This applies also to regular travellers to endemic areas — they often think they have developed immunity.

● No chemoprophylactic regimen gives total protection to everybody — warn patients that they may still contract malaria despite taking antimalarial prophylaxis.

● Consider taking drugs for standby treatment (see p. 161) as prompt medical help may not be available in the area of travel.

● Natural immunity is rapidly lost. Settled immigrants in the UK returning on visits to their home country are at risk of malaria and so they should consider chemoprophylaxis.

● Babies and pregnant women should not travel to malarious areas unless unavoidable. If they do, they must use chemoprophylaxis.

● Any febrile flu-like illness occurring in the weeks or months after travelling to a malarious area should arouse suspicion and malaria should be excluded.

● While in a malarious area seek medical advice for fever, especially if associated with rigors.

Protection against mosquito bites

● Wear long-sleeved clothing and long trousers when going out between dusk and dawn when mosquitos commonly bite. Avoid dark colours as they attract mosquitos.

● Choose air-conditioned accommodation.

● Use an insecticide spray to kill any mosquitos that may have entered the room during the day.

● Remain in well-screened areas — mosquito screens on windows, doors closed especially from late afternoon onwards.

● If mosquitos can enter during the night, use an electric mosquito killer (remember to take the appropriate adaptor to suit voltage and the sockets) or burn mosquito coils. Electronic buzzers are of no value.

● Use a mosquito net while sleeping at night, especially one that is impregnated with synthetic pyrethroids. Tuck the edges of the net under the mattress during the day so as to ensure that no mosquitos are trapped inside. Repair any holes promptly.

● Apply to exposed skin (face, hands and ankles) a mosquito repellent containing diethyl toluamide (DEET) which is available as a spray, cream, gel, stick or liquid. It may be applied to clothing. To be effective these repellents require repeated application — follow manufacturers' recommendations as they can be toxic when used in excess, especially in children.

● Consider using wrist and ankle bands impregnated with DEET. Anti-mosquito equipment can be obtained from, among others, British Airways Travel Clinics and Homeway Ltd (see p. 216).

Chemoprophylaxis
● This should be started 1 week before arrival and continued without interruption until at least 4 weeks after leaving the malarious area.

● Travellers who develop any serious side effects while taking anti-malarial chemoprophylaxis should stop it and seek medical attention.

● For infants and children the dose is calculated according to the child's weight. Breast-fed babies are not protected by their mother's prophylaxis, and require their own.

● If a pregnant woman has to travel to a malarious area, she could take proquanil (with folate supplements), chloroquine or quinine. She should not take pyrimethamine (Fansidar, Maloprim), mefloquine (Lariam), halofantrine (Halfan) or doxycycline, except on explicit medical advice.

● The use of chloroquine in patients with psoriasis may precipitate a severe attack of psoriasis. Caution should be exercised in patients with hepatic and renal disease.

● Mefloquine (Lariam) is used for travel to areas of multiple drug-resistant *P. falciparum*, such as East Africa. The prevalence of serious side effects (fits, paranoia, hallucinations and delusions, depression and severe anxiety) is low, estimated at 1 in 10 000 during prophylactic use, and 1 in 1000 when therapeutic doses are used. Some countries (not the UK) use it for travel longer than 3 months on the basis of their experience, e.g. USA Peace Corps. Do not use mefloquine in patients:

(a) with a history of convulsions (personal or immediate family);

(b) with a history of major psychiatric disorders;

(c) with renal or hepatic impairment;

(d) who are pregnant or breast-feeding or likely to become pregnant within 3 months of stopping the drug (long half-life);

(e) who undertake precision activities (e.g. airline pilots);

(f) who have concurrent administration of quinine or chloroquine;

(g) who have a history of hypersensitivity to mefloquine or quinine.

Mefloquine should not be used for standby (emergency) treatment. Separate it from oral typhoid vaccine by at least 12 h.

● We are now witnessing an increased prevalence of strains of *P. falciparum* resistant to chloroquine and proguanil. For travel to such areas another drug is added, usually mefloquine.

Table 52 Oral prophylaxis against malaria

Drug	Trade name	Tablet (base) in mg	Prophylactic dose	
			Adult	Paediatric*
Chloroquine	Avloclor Nivaquine	250 (155) 200 (150)	Two tablets once weekly	5 mg base/kg once weekly
Proguanil	Paludrine	100	Two tablets once daily	<2 years, 50 mg/day 2–6 years, 100 mg/day 7–10 years, 150 mg/day >10 years, 200 mg/day
Mefloquine	Lariam	250	One tablet once weekly	5 mg/kg once weekly (not for children under 15 kg)
Doxycycline (limited experience)	Nordox Vibramycin	100 100	One tablet daily for up to 8 weeks	Not recommended
Dapsone plus pyrimethamine	Maloprim	100 +12.5	One tablet once weekly	<5 years, not recommended 5–10 years, half a tablet >10 years, one tablet once weekly

* The paediatric dose should not exceed the adult dose.

Table 53 Children's prophylactic doses

Age	Weight	Chloroquine/ proguanil	Mefloquine	Dapsone plus pyrimethamine
0–5 weeks		1/8 adult dose	Not recommended	Not recommended
6 weeks to 1 year	Up to 10 kg	1/8–1/4 adult dose	Not recommended	Not recommended
1–5 years	10–19 kg	1/4–1/2 adult dose	< 2 years (< 15 kg) not recommended 2–5 years, 1/4 adult dose	Not recommended
6–11 years	20–39 kg	1/2–3/4 adult dose	6–8 years, 1/2 adult dose 9–11 years, 3/4 adult dose	1/2 adult dose > 10 years, one tablet
12 years to adult	> 40 kg	Adult dose	Adult dose	Adult dose

- The Malaria Reference Laboratory at the London School of Hygiene and Tropical Medicine, in collaboration with the Ross Institute, have published (*BMJ* 1993; 306; 1247–52) their recommendations on which drug or combination of drugs should be used according to country of travel. A synopsis is given here:

(a) *Malaria risk extremely low or absent.* No chemoprophylaxis but consider malaria if fever occurs in the following places:

- Algeria, Egypt, Libya, Morocco, Qatar, Tunisia, Turkey (not Anatolia);
- Bali, China (urban), Hong Kong, Indonesia (urban), Malaysia, Thailand (Bangkok and main tourist areas), Philippines (urban), Brunei;
- Cuba, Jamaica, St Lucia, Trinidad.

(b) *Malaria risk low or absent in cities.* Use chloroquine or proguanil:

- Egypt (rural, June–October), Iraq (rural, June–October), Mauritius (rural), Saudi Arabia, United Arab Emirates, Syria (rural, May– October), Turkey (Anatolia);
- Argentina (rural), Belize, Costa Rica (rural), Dominican Republic, El Salvador, Haiti, Honduras, Mexico (rural), Peru (rural).

(c) *Malaria risk high, resistance to chloroquine present.* Use chloroquine plus proguanil or mefloquine:

- Angola, Benin, Botswana, Burkina Faso, Burundi, Cameroon,

Central African Republic, Chad, Comoros, Congo, Djibouti, Equatorial Guinea, Ethiopia, Gabon, Gambia, Ghana, Guinea, Ivory Coast, Liberia, Madagascar, Mali, Mauritania, Namibia, Niger, Nigeria, Rwanda, Senegal, Sierra Leone, Somalia, South Africa (parts of Natal and Transvaal only), Sudan, Swaziland, Togo, Zimbabwe;

● Afghanistan, Bangladesh (rural), Bhutan, China (rural), India, Indonesia (rural), Iryan Jaya, Iran, Nepal (< 1500 m), Pakistan, Philippines (rural), Sri Lanka, Vietnam;

● Bolivia, Brazil (rural), Colombia, Ecuador, French Guyana, Guyana, Panama, Surinam, Venezuela (rural).

(d) *Malaria risk high, multidrug resistance.* Use mefloquine (use chloroquine plus proguanil if regimen needed for longer than 3 months, for pregnant women, for children under 2 years of age and when mefloquine is contraindicated):

● Kenya, Malawi, Mozambique, Tanzania, Uganda, Zaire, Zambia;

● Kampuchea, Thailand (borders), Burma (Mynamar).

(e) *Malaria risk high*, multidrug and *chloroquine resistance.* Use mefloquine or maloprim (dapsone and pyrimethamine) plus chloroquine: Papua New Guinea, Solomon Islands, Vanuatu.

GPs may issue an NHS prescription for antimalarial tablets for up to 3 months.

Standby (emergency) treatment

Antimalarial measures and chemoprophylaxis do not always give total protection to everybody in every part of the world. A number of travellers may, therefore, contract malaria. Some frequent travellers to endemic areas (e.g. airline flying crews) do not always take their chemoprophylaxis. In some areas prompt medical attention may not be available. Such travellers should be advised to carry with them a standby emergency treatment for use in case of fever. Quinine is the only standby drug that is completely safe for pregnant women.

Quinine (300 mg tablet)

Two tablets three times daily for 7 days *or* for 3 days followed by three tablets once of Fansidar (the second option is not for pregnant women). The children's dose for quinine is 10 mg/kg of bodyweight.

Possible side effects include tinnitus, nausea, headaches, rash and visual disturbances. Use with caution in patients with cardiac problems or G6PD deficiency. Not suitable if mefloquine is used as a prophylactic.

Fansidar (sulfadoxine 500 mg/pyrimethamine 25 mg)

Three tablets once only. The corresponding dose for children is 2–11 months, 1/4 tablet; 1–3 years, 1/2 tablet; 4–8 years, one tablet; 9–14 years, two tablets; > 14 years, three tablets. Possible side effects include rashes, insomnia, depression of haematopoiesis, Stevens–Johnson syndrome and toxic epidermal necrolysis, with a death rate around 1 in 18 000 of those using it for prophylaxis — for which it is no longer recommended. Because of growing resistance to this drug, especially in sub-Saharan Africa, it is now of limited value also as a standby treatment.

Halfan (halofantrine 250 mg)

A total of six tablets, taken two at a time, 6-hourly. Repeat course 1 week later in non-immune individuals. Children should also receive three doses (total 24 mg/kg) 6-hourly, each single dose being: 32–37 kg, one and a half tablets; 23–31 kg, one tablet; < 23 kg, appropriate dosage adjustment is not possible with the tablet presentation.

Possible side effects include nausea, vomiting, abdominal pain, diarrhoea, pruritus and rash. It is not for use in pregnancy. Because of ventricular dysrhythmias in susceptible people, WHO issued a drug alert in 1993 recommending that halofantrine should only be used as an emergency self-medication for presumptive therapy in those patients known to have normal Q-T interval. It should not be used in those with a family history of congenital Q-T prolongation, in combination with drugs or clinical conditions known to prolong Q-T interval or in patients who may suffer from thiamine deficiency, and should not be administered to patients with severe electrolyte imbalance (particularly hypokalaemia or hypomagnesaemia). Further, WHO recommends that the drug is taken on an empty stomach and should not be given in combination with mefloquine. Treatment should not exceed the recommended total dosage of 24 mg/kg bodyweight given as 8 mg/kg three times (at intervals of 6 h — maximum total dose 1500 mg).

Sources of advice on malaria

● Immunization guides are provided in some of the free medical newspapers and magazines.

● Malaria Reference Laboratory, London (0171 636 8636/636 3924). For 24-h helpline tel: 0891 600350 (payline).

- Public Health Laboratory Services London (0181 200 6868).
- Hospital for Tropical Disease, London (0171 387 4411).
- Birmingham Heartlands Hospital (0121 766 6611).
- John Radcliffe Hospital, Oxford (01865 741166).
- Manchester Monsall Hospital (0161 795 4567).
- Liverpool School of Tropical Medicine (0151 708 9393).
- Ruchill Hospital, Glasgow (0141 946 7120).
- Medical Advisory Service for Travellers Abroad (MASTA) (0891 224 100 for 24-h advice (payline)).

Footnote: At the time of going to press an important investigation in the USA was published (Lancet 1994; **343**: 1396–97). It has demonstrated prophylactic activity of azithromycin (Zithromax) against a chloroquine-resistant strain of *P. falciparum* in non-immune individuals. The investigators reported that because azithromycin eradicates the parasites in the liver before entering blood, this antibiotic could be discontinued on departure from a malarious area and still prevent disease.

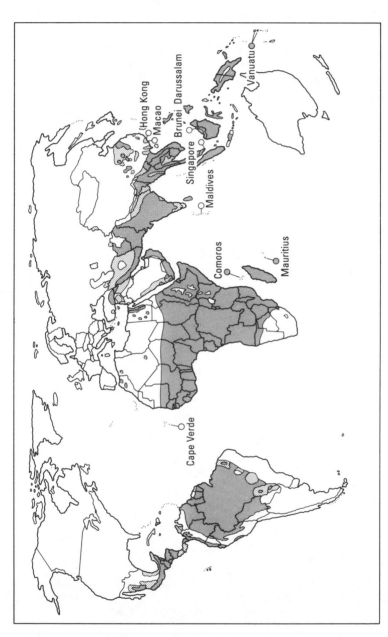

Fig. 13 Epidemiological assessment of the status of malaria, 1991. Reproduced, by permission from *Weekly Epidemiological Record* (1993, 34: 246). ☐ Areas in which malaria has disappeared or never existed; ▨ areas with limited risk; ▨ areas where malaria transmission occurs.

PRACTICAL INFORMATION

Immunization fees and the UK GP

A UK GP is an independent contractor, not a health service employee. Most of the income of British GPs derives from providing services to NHS patients and this is funded by the Department of Health (DoH).

GP earnings from immunization are derived from:

- Immunization target payments.
- Item-of-service fees for immunization.
- Direct payment by patients.

Target payments

The target payments for immunization were imposed on GPs as part of the 1990 contract. The fees payable to GPs depend on the percentage of the target population who receive the vaccinations and whether this percentage is above the targets set by the government, currently 70% vaccination uptake for the lower, and 90% for the higher, target fee. Further, these fees vary according to how much of the work is done by the GP and how much by other agencies such as immunization clinics run by health authorities.

For target payments purposes childhood immunizations are divided into two sections. The first is the percentage of children on the practice list who by the age of 2 years have achieved full group 1 (diphtheria, tetanus, polio — three doses), group 2 (pertussis — three doses) and group 3 (measles — one dose or measles/mumps/rubella (MMR) — one dose) immunization on the first day of the quarter. The second section payment is the percentage who have received boosters for diphtheria, tetanus and polio by the age of 5.

Immunization of children against *Haemophilus influenzae* type b up to the age of 50 months has attracted an item-of-service fee. Immunization of infants against *Haemophilus influenzae* b has been included in target calculations from July 1994.

Item-of-service fees

These are paid to GPs by the government only when a particular vaccination is given as a matter of public policy, either for persons remaining in this country or those travelling abroad. Fees are paid at two levels. Level B is paid for the last in a course of three or more vaccinations, or a reinforcing dose, or for vaccinations which are in a single dose. Level A fee is paid for all other vaccinations. Level B is higher than A. The following immunizations attract an item-of-service fee.

Persons not travelling abroad

- *Diphtheria and tetanus either separately or combined:* for children aged 6 years and over who have not had the basic course of immunization or a reinforcing dose. Also for staff in hospitals considered at risk of infection.
- *Tetanus:* for immunized adults (from age 15 years). For previously immunized persons having a booster on leaving school, entering higher education or starting work; thereafter, for those who have not had a booster during the previous 5 or more years.
- *Poliomyelitis:* for unimmunized 6–40 year olds, parents or guardians of children receiving oral polio, and groups at risk such as GPs, dentists, ambulance staff, GP practice staff in contact with patients, etc. For a reinforcing dose for persons aged 6 and over, and previously immunized, at school, school leaving, entering higher education or starting work and groups at risk.
- *MMR:* children not previously immunized with MMR, aged 6–15 years.
- *Measles:* children who have not previously been immunized against measles and who have not had measles, aged 6–15 years.
- *Rubella:* girls aged 10–14 years who have not previously had the MMR vaccine. Seronegative non-pregnant women of child-bearing age. Seronegative male staff working in ante-natal clinics.
- *Haemophilus influenzae b:* before the entry of Hib into the target payments in July 1994, an item-of-service fee was payable for vaccination up to the age of 50 months.
- *Infectious hepatitis:* the DoH in its *Statement of Fees and Allowances* (Red Book) does not clarify which hepatitis the term 'infectious hepatitis' covers. It is presumed to cover all types and a fee is payable for vaccinating those at risk through work and others recommended through health officers.
- *Rabies:* for groups at special risk.

Persons travelling abroad

In certain circumstances, the DoH will pay an item-of-service fee:
- *Typhoid:* travellers to an infected area or where typhoid immuni-

zation is a condition of entry. Travellers to all countries except Canada, the USA, Australia, New Zealand and northern Europe. The DoH refuses to pay a fee for the oral typhoid vaccine (self-administered by the patient) despite the fact that the patient is counselled by the GP before the vaccine is prescribed.

● *Cholera:* travellers to an infected area or where cholera immunization is a condition of entry. All travellers to Africa and Asia.

● *Poliomyelitis:* travellers to an infected area or where polio immunization is a condition of entry. Travellers to all countries except Canada, the USA, Australia, New Zealand and Europe (includes Cyprus and Turkey).

● *Infectious hepatitis:* this is assumed to refer to all types of hepatitis although the Family Health Services Authorities (FHSAs) usually pay an item-of-service fee for the administration of hepatitis A gammaglobulin. Some will pay the fee for a full course of the vaccine. FHSAs differ in their interpretation of payments for hepatitis A vaccine. For persons travelling outside northern Europe, Australia and New Zealand who are going to reside for 3 months or longer, or who, if infected, might be less resistant because of pre-existing disease, or who are travelling to areas of poor sanitation.

Direct payments

Such payments are only allowed from non-NHS (private) patients. Also from NHS patients travelling abroad where their vaccination is not covered by the *Statement of Fees and Allowances.* An example is yellow fever immunization. GPs are also allowed to charge NHS patients requesting international vaccination certificates.

Notes

Personal dispensing of vaccines by GPs

Non-dispensing GPs in England and Wales can claim a fee for purchasing and dispensing available vaccines under paragraph 44.5 of the *Statement of Fees and Allowances*. The vaccines may be administered by the doctor or the practice nurse. Overall, the government reimburses the GP the drug tariff basic price of the vaccine with an additional on-cost allowance of 10.5%, a container allowance, a dispensing fee and an allowance in respect of value added tax. Obtaining a discount from the supplier increases the practice profit. This scheme allows practices to organize many immunization campaigns such as the annual influenza vaccination programme, that do not attract an item-of-service fee.

Not all vaccines are available for GPs to purchase. Vaccines for childhood immunizations are supplied directly to health authorities and GPs by the DoH appointed distributors. These include *Haemophilus influenzae* b, MMR, rubella, BCG, diphtheria, DTP, DT, pertussis, polio and tuberculin-purified protein derivative. Before purchasing vaccines, the GP is well advised to check with his or her local Family Health Service Authority or the Prescription Pricing Authority, as to whether the particular vaccine is available under the scheme.

Notes

Immunization and the practice audit

Audit is a systematic way of looking critically at the work that GPs are involved in to see if changing it could lead to an improvement. It is a useful tool by which GPs can check what they are doing is what they think they ought to be doing, and what improvements can be made.

Audit can be very well applied to immunization. You may, for example, want to see whether all patients for whom annual influenza vaccination is recommended, do indeed receive the vaccine. Audit will measure the practice performance with regard to the influenza campaign. Such an audit will not only show how well (or badly) the practice is doing but will also stimulate discussion among the members of the primary health-care team, encourage change (if it is required) and allow for reassessment of changes by being repeated every year.

Here is an example of an audit the practice could adopt or modify with regard to influenza immunization. It can be modified to cover any other immunization.

The audit method

- *The rationale:* patients at risk of complications from contracting influenza because of their medical condition or age could benefit from annual influenza immunization.
- *The aim*: to examine whether all patients for whom the DoH recommends annual influenza immunization have received the vaccine this year.

Criteria

The proposed criteria relate to patients for whom the DoH recommends annual influenza immunization. Patients with the following conditions/ situations should have received the vaccine during the last 12 months:

- Chronic heart disease.
- Chronic respiratory disease, including asthma.
- Chronic renal disease.
- Diabetes mellitus.
- Other endocrine conditions.

- Immunosuppression due to disease or treatment.
- People living in residential homes.

A practice may wish to recommend influenza immunization to otherwise healthy individuals over 65 years of age, as is recommended in the USA. If so, this group of patients could make up another criterion to be looked at.

Standard

That 80% of these patients should have received the influenza vaccine this year (choose other standard if you wish).

Methods of data collection

- Nominate members of staff to carry out the audit, meet with them and explain the aims and proceedings.
- If you adopt the criterion that patients above 65 will be in the target group, identify them through the practice computer or the age–sex register.
- Identify patients with various conditions by the practice disease register or repeat prescriptions, opportunistic surgery attendance, health promotion or disease clinics, over-75 checks and personal memory (doctor, nurse and staff). Patients in homes can be identified by their addresses.
- Ideally you will wish to include in this audit all your patients in the target group but this will probably not be possible because of the numbers. Select an appropriate size for a representative sample — excellent details of choosing a sample are given in the magazine *Managing Audit in General Practice* (1993; 1(2): 17–20).
- Scrutinize each set of notes to determine the presence or absence of flu vaccine administration this year (October–April) and transfer information on spread sheets or a specially written computer programme.
- Interrogate the computer if all flu vaccinations are on it.
- Agree on a reasonable timescale for completion of data collection.
- Prepare the data for analysis by collating the information on computer or data evaluation sheets (Table 54).

Compare performance with standards

Have at least 80% of patients with chronic conditions as recommended by the DoH, or have at least 80% of patients aged 65 and above (if this was also your criterion), received the influenza vaccine this year?

Table 54 Example of a data evaluation sheet

No	Name	Date of birth	Sex	Flu vaccine (Y/N)	Date (month/year)
1	Smith, PA	2.5.25	M	Y	Oct. 1992
2	Taylor, JA	2.8.13	F	N	—
3	Patel, P	11.3.19	F	N	—
4	Wallace, AN	19.11.03	M	Y	Nov. 1992
5	Ryan, T	6.3.15	F	Y	Oct. 1992
6	Roberts, NY	4.11.05	M	Y	Jan. 1993
7	Alexander, JN	6.8.09	M	N	—
8	Morris, AC	30.9.14	F	N	—
9	Marsh, TS	26.2.26	F	Y	Dec. 1992

If you have not achieved your set standards, decide on a course of action. You may decide that you will plan your next influenza campaign early, order your vaccines early, organize nurse-run influenza vaccination clinics or increase the number of such clinics, write to your target patients, attach to the repeat prescriptions a letter of invitation to an influenza vaccination clinic, put posters in the waiting room, personally (and your partners) promote immunization against influenza, and so on.

Remeasure your performance annually by repeating this audit.

Notes

The practice nurse and immunization*

Part of the work of the practice nurse is to promote the benefits of, and to carry out, immunization. In most circumstances, immunization is an elective procedure particularly for young children. The vaccines used to immunize children against infectious diseases are among the safest drugs available, provided their contraindications are observed.

It is important to understand the difference between immunization and vaccination, as these two terms are often used interchangeably in practice. To immunize is to make immune, especially by inoculation, whereas to vaccinate is to inoculate (a person) with vaccine so as to produce immunity against a specific disease. Immunity is an intrinsic or acquired state of resistance to an infectious agent. Natural immunity is acquired following infection and the subsequent production of anti-bodies, whereas immunization is achieved following the administration of antigens by inoculation, to stimulate the production of antibodies and induce immunity artificially. Therefore, vaccination is the act of vaccinating against a disease with immunization being the acquisition of immunity to the disease.

Although the immediate goal is the prevention of infectious disease in the individual and the community, the ultimate objective is eradication. In countries with successful immunization programmes, virtual elimination of tetanus, diphtheria, poliomyelitis, pertussis, measles, mumps and rubella is being observed.

An essential part of the role of the practice nurse is to understand fully the reasons for immunization, contraindications, adverse reactions and special precautions indicated for each infectious disease. Most of the necessary descriptive and factual background is contained within this book; it is important that this information is used, coupled with the nurse's teaching and counselling abilities, to promote a healthy practice population.

Protocols for immunization must be agreed by the GP, practice nurse and other team members to ensure both safety and high standards

* This section on 'The Practice Nurse' appeared first in the distance-learning tutorial the author wrote for the series *Magister*.

of practice. Whilst the practice nurse should encourage immunization at all times, there must be respect for individual choice and patients or parents should not be cajoled into vaccination against their wishes. A better approach would be to explain and discuss the risks of refusal of immunization.

The GP contract (April, 1990) introduced target payments for childhood immunizations, with 70% achievement as the lower target and 90% as the higher target. Practice nurses should familiarize themselves with the statutory changes which take place from time to time in immunization programmes.

Most importantly, the practice nurse should promote immunization in the community and carry out successful immunization campaigns. No child should be denied immunization. To deny a child immunization may be to deny that child good health.

Medicolegal aspects of immunization and the nurse

The practice nurse has two main responsibilities in the administration of vaccines to a patient. The first of these responsibilities is to ensure his or her own competence in undertaking the activity, and the second is to ensure that the correct vaccine is given to the right patient and in the correct circumstances. These responsibilities are, of course, not mutually exclusive. Following the administration of any vaccine, patients should remain at the surgery for a further 20 min for observation for adverse reactions.

Following through the guiding principles associated with any activity, the nurse giving a vaccine must have had specific and adequate training to carry out the procedure; his or her employing GP must be satisfied with the competence of the nurse, and of course the nurse must feel that he or she is equipped and competent to undertake this exercise.

The nurse who gives any vaccine must have a thorough knowledge of that vaccine, its correct dosage, route of administration, adverse effects, contraindications and compatibility. The nurse must also be able to recognize and treat an anaphylactic shock reaction. Only when these criteria have been met should the nurse be involved in immunization procedures.

Having established the appropriate knowledge base the nurse needs to give due regard to the 'legal' processes which govern the administration of medicines. It is recommended that nurses refer to the advisory paper 'United Kingdom Central Council for Nurses, Midwives and Health Visitors, Administration of Medicines' (UKCC, 1986).

The most obvious point is that, at present, nurses are not in a position to prescribe immunizations themselves; as such the nurse will have to establish that a prescription originated by the GP is in existence.

This prescription can be in the form of an instruction in an individual's notes or record card, or may take the form of a 'group protocol'.

This latter form of prescription — the 'protocol prescription' — is probably the most common means by which a practice nurse will operate an immunization clinic and has been accepted as an appropriate method by the UKCC as part of their 'Statement on practice nurses and aspects of a new GP contract (1990)':

> In order to ensure that the interests of patients are best served it is essential that ... any forms of medication, under current prescribing arrangements, are individually prescribed in advance by medical practitioners or are the subject of a local protocol approved by all the medical practitioners concerned and which is acceptable to the nurses involved. (1990, 3: 52)

One further step which should be followed through before giving any vaccine, is to ascertain the informed consent of the patient receiving the dose, or in the case of a child, the consent of the responsible adult.

Providing that the practice nurse adheres to these principles, he or she will be able to offer a comprehensive high quality immunization/vaccination service to patients within the practice population.

Notes

Pregnancy and immunization

Live viral vaccines

Yellow fever. Vaccine not recommended in pregnancy unless travel to areas of high risk is unavoidable. In such cases vaccination should be considered as the risk to the mother of yellow fever infection may far outweigh the small theoretical risk of fetal infection from the vaccine.

Measles. Should not be given during pregnancy and 3 (minimum 1) months before. May be given in the postpartum period.

Rubella. Should not be given during pregnancy and 1 month before. May be given in the postpartum period.

Oral poliomyelitis. Should be avoided in pregnancy especially during the first 16 weeks, unless there is a high risk of infection to the mother.

Live bacterial vaccines

Tuberculosis (BCG). Should be avoided particularly in the early stages and if possible be delayed until after delivery. However, where there is a significant risk of infection, the importance of vaccination may outweigh the possible risk to the fetus.

Typhoid (oral). Avoid (no data), unless the mother is at risk.

Inactivated viral vaccines

Influenza. Should not normally be given in pregnancy unless there is a specific risk, although there is no evidence that inactivated influenza vaccine causes damage to the fetus.

Poliomyelitis (injectable). Should be avoided unless there is an increased risk to the mother.

Hepatitis A. Not recommended in pregnancy unless there is a very definite risk of hepatitis A infection, in which case vaccination should not be withheld.

Rabies. Pre-exposure vaccine should only be given in pregnancy if the risk of exposure to rabies is high.

Tick-borne encephalitis. May be given in pregnancy if indicated.

Japanese B encephalitis. The manufacturer does not recommend the vaccine in pregnancy unless there is a definite risk of infection.

Inactivated bacterial vaccines

Typhoid (whole cell). Should be avoided unless there is a definite risk of infection.

Cholera. Should be avoided in pregnancy unless there is a definite risk of infection. The vaccine is less protective than typhoid, and cholera is rarely caught by travellers. It is, therefore, best avoided in pregnancy.

Pertussis. Avoid, unless a young unimmunized mother is at high risk.

Toxoids

Tetanus. May be used in pregnancy if necessary.

Diphtheria. Avoid in pregnancy (no data available) unless the mother is at increased risk.

Bioengineered

Hepatitis B. Not recommended in pregnancy unless there is a very definite risk of hepatitis B infection, in which case vaccination should not be withheld.

Polysaccharide extracts

Haemophilus influenzae b. Avoid (not data available).

Meningococcal A and C. Avoid unless the mother is at risk.

Pneumococcal. Avoid (no data). If a pregnant woman is at high risk, if possible wait until after first trimester of pregnancy.

Vi typhoid. Avoid, unless the mother is at risk.

Notifiable diseases

Notifiable diseases in England and Wales	Notifiable diseases in Northern Ireland	Notifiable diseases in Scotland
Acute encephalitis	Acute encephalitis	Anthrax
Acute meningitis	Acute meningitis	Chickenpox
Acute poliomyelitis	Anthrax	Cholera
Anthrax	Cholera	Diphtheria
Cholera	Diphtheria	Bacillary dysentery
Diphtheria	Dysentery	Food poisoning
Dysentery (amoebic or bacillary)	Food poisoning (all sources)	Legionellosis
Food poisoning (all sources)	Gastroenteritis (persons under 2 years of age only)	Leptospirosis
Leprosy	Infective hepatitis	Malaria
Leptospirosis	Lassa fever	Measles
Malaria	Marburg disease	Membranous croup
Measles	Paratyphoid fever	Meningooccal infection
Meningoccal septicaemia (without meningitis)	Plague	Mumps
Mumps	Poliomyelitis: paralytic and non-paralytic	Paratyphoid fever
Ophthalmia neonatorum	Rabies	Puerperal fever
Paratyphoid fever	Relapsing fever	Rabies
Plague	Scarlet fever	Relapsing fever
Rabies	Smallpox	Rubella
Relapsing fever	Tuberculosis: pulmonary and non-pulmonary	Scarlet fever
Rubella	Typhoid fever	Smallpox
Scarlet fever	Typhus	Tetanus
Smallpox	Viral haemorrhagic fever	Tuberculosis
Tetanus	Whooping cough	Typhoid fever
Tuberculosis	Yellow fever	Typhus fever
Typhoid fever		Viral haemorrhagic fever
Typhus		Viral hepatitis
Viral haemorrhagic fever		Whooping cough
Viral hepatitis		
Whooping cough		
Yellow fever		

- A fee is payable to doctors in the UK who notify any of the above diseases. The average GP notifies fewer than 12 infectious diseases each year and this is considered to be underreporting.
- Acquired immune deficiency syndrome (AIDS) is not a notifiable disease in the UK. Nonetheless, doctors are advised to report new cases to the Director, PHLS Communicable Disease Surveillance Centre, London.

Notes

Information sheet for parents

(This data may be copied and given to parents.)

● Immunization is the process of making a person resistant to a disease without suffering its symptoms. This is usually achieved by inoculation (injecting vaccine into the body) or by drops (oral polio vaccine).

● Immunization of a child not only protects that child but it helps prevent the infectious diseases from spreading to the rest of the family and the community.

● Vaccines usually give well over 90% protection if a full course of immunization is given. If a vaccinated child still catches the disease, he or she will usually have a mild form.

● Before having your child immunized, ask yourself:

(a) Is my child ill with a raised temperature?

(b) Has my child reacted to any previous immunization?

(c) Has my child ever had any kind of fits or convulsions?

(d) Does my child react to eggs or any antibiotics with a rash, swelling of the mouth and throat, difficulty in breathing and collapse?

If your answer to any of these questions is yes, or if you are unsure, talk

Table 55 Timetable for routine immunization

Age	Vaccine
2 months	Diphtheria, tetanus, whooping cough, polio, *Haemophilus influenzae* b
3 months	Diphtheria, tetanus, whooping cough, polio, *Haemophilus influenzae* b
4 months	Diphtheria, tetanus, whooping cough, polio, *Haemophilus influenzae* b
12–18 months	Measles/mumps/rubella (MMR)
4–5 years	Diphtheria, tetanus, polio
Girls 10–14 years	Rubella (if MMR not previously given)
13 years	Tuberculosis (BCG)
15–19 years	Diphtheria, tetanus, polio

it over with your doctor. He or she may advise postponement or avoidance of a particular vaccine.

● Allergies such as eczema, asthma or hay fever are not contra-indications to immunizations. Some vaccines contain traces of some antibiotics, hen's egg, etc. These vaccines are contraindicated in children who experience an anaphylactic reaction (swelling of the upper airways, collapse) and not just a dislike or rash when they ingest these antibiotics, hen's eggs, etc.

● Your child needs to be immunized against measles, mumps and rubella even if you think your child has already had one or more of these diseases. This is because there are many childhood illnesses which look like measles or German measles, so it is impossible to be sure that your child has indeed had them.

● If your child has already received the measles or rubella (German measles) vaccine, your doctor may suggest to you that your child receives the M M R combined vaccine. There is no harm in being immunized twice against measles or rubella even if your child has already had one of these diseases before, and the M M R vaccine will also give your child protection against mumps.

● If your child has not been immunized and comes into contact with a child with measles, he or she can still be protected if the M M R vaccine is given within 3 days of contact.

● If your child vomits within 1 h of receiving the oral polio vaccine, a further dose is necessary.

Reactions to vaccines

● All medicines have some risks but the vaccines used to immunize children against infectious diseases are among the safest.

● The infectious diseases themselves can cause the same problems as the vaccines. The risk of harmful side effects from vaccines is a lot smaller than from infectious diseases.

● Many children for whom immunization is perfectly safe can experience mild, harmless side effects. A child might cry a bit more than usual, become slightly feverish and irritable for a few hours after the injection. Some children show some redness and swelling at the site of the injection. Some children may get fever and a measles rash 5–10 days after receiving the M M R combined vaccine. The rash lasts for 2–3 days and it is not transmissible to unvaccinated children. Occasionally a child may develop swollen glands on the face like mumps, about 3 or more weeks after vaccination with M M R. Others may complain of joint aches.

● The chances of more serious side effects are very rare indeed, and they occur much less frequently after immunization than if the child was to catch the disease. Febrile convulsions after measles disease are eight to 10 times more common than after the measles vaccine. If brain damage from whooping cough vaccine occurs at all, it occurs so rarely that it is difficult to prove. In fact, whooping cough vaccine may be protecting your child from brain damage by preventing whooping cough disease which may be complicated by brain damage.

● If your child has a tendency to convulsions, you should discuss with the doctor the management of any fever and/or convulsions possibly developing after immunization. This could happen in the first 72 h after whooping cough immunization or 5–10 days after M M R immunization. In case of fever, it is recommended that you give the baby paracetamol, extra fluids, dress them in thin clothing, cool the room and even perform tepid sponging and consider having the child seen by the GP.

● Children receiving their oral polio vaccine can continue excreting the vaccine virus in their faeces for up to 6 months after vaccination. We would recommend adherence to strict personal hygiene for anybody who changes the nappies and in particular washing hands after nappy changes and safe disposal of the nappies. If any member of the family has not been immunized against polio, they should also receive the vaccine at the same time as the baby.

● Please report to the doctor any symptoms your child experiences after immunization that worry you.

● To deny vaccination can be to deny the child its health. Your help in protecting your child and all children against infectious diseases is greatly appreciated and welcomed.

Notes

TRAVEL AND IMMUNIZATION

Travel clinics

We are now witnessing a boom in international travel. In 1948 world airlines transported 4 000 000 international passengers — in 1990 that figure rose to 1 160 000 000, of which 31 000 000 were UK residents.

GPs and practice nurses have an important role in giving people both general and specific advice about travel abroad. Further, they have the responsibility of recognizing diseases 'imported' from abroad, and treating those returning unwell. Travel medicine has, therefore, become established as a speciality area within the general practice setting. The contribution of practice nurses has become invaluable as many of them run the travel clinics under the guidance of the GPs they work with.

It is important to note that less than 50% of travel-related illness is currently preventable by vaccines and that the commonest illnesses acquired abroad are preventable by measures other than immunization.

In general, 'low-risk' travellers are holiday-makers or business people staying in high standard hotels or major cities. 'High-risk' travellers are health-care personnel and others going to work or stay for a considerable time or to live in developing countries.

It should be emphasized to travellers that immunization against infectious diseases does not give complete protection. The importance of good personal precautions should be stressed, such as care over eating and drinking, avoiding insect and animal bites and sensible personal contact and hygiene.

Legal aspects of advice for travellers

Published recommendations should be followed carefully. A decision not to follow such advice should be documented in the notes with reasons and warnings given.

The Medical Defence Union's advice to GPs states: 'There must be a very real possibility of a claim for negligence being made against a doctor who deliberately overrides a country's recommendations and the patient contracts one of the specified diseases. It is likely to prove extremely difficult to mount an adequate defence against this claim'.

After due consideration if a doctor genuinely feels vaccination is contraindicated, he or she should provide the patient with a certificate giving full details of the reasons for non-vaccination. In such cases an airline may permit travel but it is the health authority at the port of arrival which is the final arbiter on those arriving without valid certificates where they are required. Such travellers may be liable to inconvenience, delay and even quarantine at their final destination. Some risk having to receive vaccination at the border, sometimes with needles of questionable sterility.

For product liability purposes, the batch number of all vaccines/immunoglobulins should be recorded in the patient's notes. Vaccines should be stored under the conditions recommended by the manufacturers, usually at refrigerator temperatures of between $+2$ and $+8°C$ (best at $3°$ to $4°C$). Unused reconstituted vaccines or used multidose vials should be discarded after a vaccination session.

Another area with medicolegal implications is the doctor offering help to a patient on a flight. Under American law, a doctor who attends a patient during an in-flight emergency, could be sued where the aircraft is registered or where it is owned, where the incident took place, where the plaintiff lives, where the defendant lives or even, on some occasions, in more than one place at once.

General advice

● *Sensible eating and drinking.* Gastrointestinal problems, predominantly diarrhoea and vomiting, are the major cause of illness for travellers abroad. Give advice on how to avoid these problems as well as what to do with some medications in the case of diarrhoea and vomiting — this applies particularly to patients on diuretics and angiotensin-converting enzyme inhibitors where diarrhoea can lead to dehydration and kidney failure.

● *Road traffic and other accidents.* Warn patients that more Britons die abroad in road traffic accidents or by drowning than due to all immunizable diseases added together.

● *Alcohol, sea and sun warnings.* Sensible alcohol intake. Gradual exposure to the sun, wearing a hat and sunglasses, filter suncreams, and avoidance of direct sun between 11 a.m. and 2 p.m. Avoidance of contact with jellyfish.

● *Safer sex.* Inappropriate sexual behaviour abroad increases the risk of contracting HIV 300-fold. Apart from HIV, travellers could contract herpes, syphilis, gonorrhoea and chlamydia.

● *Contact with animals.* Avoid any contact, especially with stray or wild animals.

- *Antimalaria prophylaxis*. Lack of it increases the traveller's chance of dying from malaria 20-fold.
- *Combating stress*. Travellers may be subject to various forms of stress, such as overcrowding, long hours of waiting, changes in climate and time zones, and disruption of eating habits. They need to plan ahead and allow sufficient time for journeys. They also need to plan when they are going to take their prescribed medications, such as insulin or diuretics. Stress and problems with medication contribute to the fact that cardiovascular disease is the most frequent cause of death occurring abroad in travellers aged 50–70 years. They should take adequate supplies of their prescribed medication and should not put all supplies in the baggage hold as baggage can be delayed or lost.
- *Medical kit*. It is sensible to take one, especially if travelling to a remote destination. Sterile medical packs, which contain syringes, needles, injection swabs, drip needle for blood transfusion, needle set for stitching, skin closure strips, dressings and gloves, are available commercially from travel clinics, some pharmacies and from organizations such as Homeway Ltd (01962 881526).
- *Mosquito nets*. Obtainable from the above sources.
- *Adequate medical insurance*. This is essential, particularly in the USA. The traveller should ensure that his or her medical condition, e.g. diabetes, is not excluded in the policy. If travelling to an EEC country, the traveller should take Form E111 fully completed and stamped at the post office. Some non-EEC countries have reciprocal health-care agreements with the UK.
- *Health Care Advice for Travellers*, a DoH publication, can be obtained free from the DoH (0800 555777).

Air travel
Reduction of alveolar pressure of oxygen at high altitudes during aircraft travel can result in desaturation of arterial blood by about 3%. Patients with conditions such as heart failure, ischaemic heart disease, cerebral artery insufficiency, respiratory disease or severe anaemia may have problems because of this and may need extra oxygen.

Contraindications to air travel
(as advised by the British Airways Health Services)
- Severe anaemia.
- Severe cases of sinusitis and otitis media.
- Acute contagious or communicable disease.

- Recent myocardial infarction.
- Uncontrolled cardiac failure.
- Recent cerebral infarction.
- Peptic ulceration — within 3 weeks of haemorrhage.
- Postoperative cases — within 10 days of simple abdominal operation; and within 14 days of major chest surgery.
- Skin diseases which are contagious or repulsive in appearance.
- Fractures of the mandible with fixed wiring of the jaw.
- Mental illness without escort and sedation.
- Within 7 days of introduction of air to body cavities for diagnostic or therapeutic purposes.
- Terminally ill patients unlikely to survive the journey.

Traveller's diarrhoea

This occurs in up to 50% of travellers abroad. It is nearly always contracted from contaminated food or water. Contamination is usually from a food handler who is a faecal carrier, from uncooked or unwashed vegetables or fruit that has been contaminated with human faeces, and also from milk from infected animals. Contamination is usually due to inadequate human sewage disposal and sometimes directly from animals. Swimming pools can be a source of infection if chlorination is inadequate. Some water-borne organisms enter the body through the skin, for example schistosomiasis and hookworm. Sometimes, diarrhoea may be due to dietary indiscretions.

The most common causative agents are:

- Gram-negative bacteria, such as *Escherichia coli*, some strains of *Salmonella*, *Shigella*, *Vibrio cholerae* and *Campylobacter*.
- Protozoa such as *Entamoeba histolytica*, *Giardia lamblia* and *Cryptosporidium*.
- Viruses, such as Rotavirus, enteric adenovirus, astrovirus, calcivirus and the Norwalk virus.
- Toxins such as staphylococcal and clostridial toxins.

Although the condition is usually self-limiting, dehydration is particularly dangerous in elderly people, especially for those on diuretics. For mild cases, a finger pinch of salt and a teaspoonful of sugar in 250 ml of water is an effective mixture. More severe cases require proprietary electrolyte solutions such as Dioralyte, Rehidrat or Electrolade.

Administration of antidiarrhoeal drugs such as loperamide (Imodium) or diphenoxylate (Lomotil) should not be undertaken routinely. Antibiotics are sometimes indicated (quinolones, erythromycin).

Advice to prevent diarrhoea

- Drink only reputable brands of bottled water, otherwise boil the water you drink or use to wash and brush your teeth. Avoid ice in drinks.
- Meat and vegetables should be properly cooked and served hot.
- Avoid milk, unless well boiled — beware of milk products such as cream, cheeses and ice cream.

- Avoid salads and fruit that may be washed in suspect water. Choose vegetables and fruit that can be peeled, such as bananas, melons, papaya or avocado.
- Avoid raw fish and shellfish.
- Avoid food from street vendors — eat only in reputable places.

The diabetic traveller*

Before setting off

Vaccinations

Diabetic patients should ensure they have all the required vaccinations for the countries they are going to visit. Diabetes itself is not a contra-indication to vaccination, and diabetics are no more or less likely to contract illnesses abroad. On the other hand, if they become ill the consequences could be more serious than in non-diabetics.

Immunization may be followed by a day or two of feeling unwell as a result of a local or systemic reaction. There can be a temporary rise of blood sugar. These problems are rarely of any concern.

If travelling to an area where malaria is endemic, the patient should remember to start appropriate anti-malarial tablets 1 week before departure and continue to take them until at least 4 weeks after leaving that area.

Insurance

The diabetic patient may require hospital or other medical care while abroad, be it as a result of accident, the diabetes or some other illness, and treatment may be very expensive. In addition, the diabetic patient may have to cancel his or her holiday for a reason beyond his or her control or as a result of illness. Comprehensive travel insurance that does not exclude diabetes or a pre-existing illness must be obtained. For UK residents Form E111 will enable the diabetic patient to get emergency medical care within the European Union (EU) for short stays of less than 1 year (the forms are available from post offices or Department of Social Security local offices). Some non-EU countries also have reciprocal health-care agreements with the UK.

Medical supplies

Adequate supplies of medication should be packed so that the patient

---

* This section on diabetes and travel appeared first in an article the author wrote for *Diabetes Reviews International* (1994; 3(2): 11–13) published by Macmillan Magazines.

does not run short and is able to replace lost items. Two or three times the estimated requirements of supplies should normally be taken to cover such emergencies. This applies not only to insulin or oral hypo-glycaemics but also to blood glucose testing strips, urine glucose and ketone testing strips, finger-pricking devices and lancets, insulin syringes, glucagon, glucose tablets and needle disposal container (in an emergency a soft drink can will do).

For longer stays, the diabetic patient should make arrangements for continuous supplies of insulin abroad. Some larger pharmacies can send insulin abroad by prior arrangement if there is no suitable insulin in the country of destination. In Europe many countries still have insulin 40 rather than 100 units ml strength. If the patient runs out of U-100 and gets U-40 insulin, he or she should be instructed to ask for U-40 syringes so that the lines on the syringe will correspond to the units of insulin. Countries that use U-40 insulin include France, Germany, Italy, Spain, Yugoslavia, the Czech and Slovak Republics, Morocco, Russia, Tunisia, Algeria, Kenya, Nigeria, Egypt, Syria, China, Japan and Korea.

Transporting and storing insulin

Insulin will remain stable, even if partly used for up to 2 years or more (depending on the expiry date) if stored in a refrigerator, which normally has a temperature of 2–8°C. Insulin should not be stored in or close to the freezer compartment, as freezing will damage it, with loss of effectiveness. Exposing the vials to sunlight or high temperature will do similar damage.

If kept below room temperature (20–25°C), insulin will remain stable for up to 1 month. If travelling for longer or to particularly hot or cold parts of the world, patients should carry their insulin in a polystyrene container or a wide-necked vacuum flask which can be rinsed out with cold water or ice in the morning. Alternatively, if freezer facilities are available, an insulated storage bag with a frozen plastic insert can be used, but the vials of insulin should not come in contact with the frozen plastic container in case the insulin freezes.

A frequent visual check of the insulin should be made. If soluble insulin looks cloudy or 'clumpy' in appearance it should be discarded. Isophane, Lente and pre-mixed insulins normally have a cloudy appearance. When such insulin is damaged, the cloudiness is uneven, with solidified pieces appearing as clumps when the vial is gently rotated. Sometimes damaged insulin takes on a brownish colour.

Other considerations before setting off

Storage of glucagon should pose no problem, as it comes as a powder with a vial of water for dilution. The patient should bear in mind that some blood glucose testing strips over-read in very hot climates and under-read in extreme cold. (Check with manufacturers.)

The patient should carry identification in the form of a bracelet, pendant, disc or identification card of a letter from the patient's physician stating the tablet or insulin dosage and the patient's details. Moreover, the address and telephone number of the diabetic association in the country of destination and the nearest hospital to the resort should be noted.

Some Muslim countries may not allow use of porcine insulin. The patient should check with the appropriate embassy, preferably in writing, and, if it is necessary and possible, the patient should change to human insulin well before departure.

The inclusion of a medical kit, sun cream, sun hat and mosquito nets in the luggage, as appropriate, is advisable. Travel guides from diabetic associations will provide details about food and other important information for many tourist destinations.

During the journey

Journeys can be unexpectedly delayed. The diabetic patient should carry emergency snacks for such eventualities. If prone to travel sickness, medication to prevent it should be taken. When passing through customs the patient may be required to account for needles and syringes he or she is carrying. Airport X-ray machines will not damage insulin.

Luggage

Insulin and testing equipment should not be packed in suitcases. Aeroplanes fly at altitudes that can cause freezing in the baggage hold. In addition, baggage can be delayed or lost. Insulin and testing equipment should, therefore, be packed in hand-held luggage.

Immobility

Long journeys on buses, trains or aeroplanes can cause feet to swell and predispose to leg thrombosis because of the enforced immobility. The diabetic patient should, therefore, be advised to walk up and down the aisle whenever possible and to take some comfortable shoes or slippers to wear on the journey.

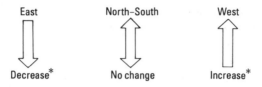

Fig. 14 Insulin dose change when travelling
* By 2–4% of daily dose of insulin per hour of time shift

Adjustments of insulin dose and monitoring

Travelling across several time zones changes a patient's schedule for insulin injections (Fig. 14). As a general rule the international traveller needs to increase his or her dose of insulin when travelling west and decrease it when travelling east. Frequent monitoring by blood testing, at least every 6 h is advisable. There is no need to adjust insulin for north–south travel. Generally, it is necessary to increase or decrease by 2–4% the daily dose of insulin for each hour of time shift for each westward or eastward flight (Table 56).

For westward travel the shift in time zone should be covered by one or two extra injections of short-acting insulin on the plane. The additional dose is 20– 30% of the total daily dose (2–4% per time-shift hour).

For eastward travel, the late evening meal on the plane is covered with an extra dose of short-acting insulin (2–6 units). The subsequent breakfast dose of intermediate-acting insulin should be reduced by 20– 40% (3–5% per time-shift hour), but the usual dose of short-acting insulin can be injected. The late timing (in local time) of the morning

Table 56 Insulin dose changes

Going west (longer day)
Extra short-acting insulin on the plane
–2–4% per time-shift hour (one or two doses)

Going east (shorter day)
Short-acting insulin (2–6 units) for late evening meal on flight
Breakfast dose on arrival:
- On short-acting insulin: no change
- On intermediate-acting insulin: reduce dose by 3–5% per time-shift hour
- If on lunchtime dose too: omit it

Adapted from Sane *et al.* (*Br Med J* 1990; 301: 421–2).

Table 57 Dose of insulin if crossing six or more time zones

Going west Check glucose 18 h after morning dose — if elevated, give extra insulin
Going east Reduce regular insulin dose by a third Check glucose 10 h later — if elevated, give extra insulin

Adapted from Benson *et al.* (*Bull Mason Clinic* 1984–1985; 38: 145–51).

injection means that an injection before lunch is not necessary in patients who normally have one.

Another formula for insulin dose readjustment is for westbound travellers who cross six or more time zones to adjust their insulin dose for the longer day (Table 57). If the blood glucose is elevated 18 h after the morning injection, an extra dose of insulin is given. For eastbound travel, adjustment should be made for the shortened day. The regular insulin dose should be reduced to two-thirds on the first morning of arrival (at local time); testing and readjusting the dose should be carried out 10 h later if the blood glucose is elevated.

Patients an oral hypoglycaemics could consider staying on home time for medication and meals until they can adjust on arrival.

Alcohol should be avoided while travelling as it can lead to dehydration.

At the destination

Physical activity
This increases the likelihood of hypoglycaemia, so diabetic patients may need to increase carbohydrate intake. Inactivity while lying on the beach all day and overeating may increase blood glucose and this can be compensated for by extra insulin. On the other hand, the absorption of insulin in hot climates is faster and can precipitate hypoglycaemia. In such situations frequent blood test monitoring should be carried out.

Walking barefoot on hot sand and other trauma to the feet should be avoided.

Fluids and food
In some countries it may not be safe to drink the local tap water, so sterilizing tablets or bottled water are recommended. Adequate fluid

intake should be ensured. Alcohol can be dangerous in hot, humid climates and can lead to dehydration. Fruit and vegetables should be washed in sterilized or bottle water if the local water is suspect. Avoid adding ice to drinks in such circumstances.

Illness, infection and accidents

Most problems arise from ingestion of contaminated food or water. In the case of vomiting and/or diarrhoea the diabetic traveller should be advised not to stop taking his or her insulin or tablets but to monitor blood glucose levels frequently and adjust the insulin dose accordingly. Solid food and milk should be substituted with carbohydrate-containing proprietary salt and sugar solution. In an emergency, a solution can be made by mixing 1 level teaspoonful of salt and 8 level teaspoonfuls of sugar in 1 litre of water. If vomiting/or diarrhoea persists, medical advice should be sought.

By following relatively simple rules and careful planning there are no reasons why a diabetic patient cannot have just as enjoyable a holiday abroad as anyone else.

Disabled travellers

Increasing numbers of people with disabilities are making journeys, travelling either independently or with tour operators. Those who have done it before are usually confident but the newly disabled person may lack confidence to travel for fear of embarrassment or the unknown. Such travellers will find these sources of information helpful:

- Another disabled person who has travelled before.
- Publications such as *Holiday, Disabled Traveller* by Alison Walsh (written for the BBC *Holiday* programme) and *Nothing Ventured: disabled people travel the world*, Penguin Books (1991).
- Organizations such as the Royal Association for Disability and Rehabilitation (0171 250 3222) and Tripscope (0117 9414 094).
- Air Transport Users Committee, Care in the Air gives advice for handicapped travellers (0171 242 3882).

Notes

Sources of travel information for GPs

- Reference charts that appear regularly in medical newspapers and magazines.
- *Health Care Advice for Travellers* (DoH) (tel: 0800 555 777).
- Department of Health (0171 210 3000)
- Evans Vaccines Information — medical information (01372 364100) and 24-h advice line (01625 537607).
- Merieux Vaccination Information Service (01628 773737).
- SmithKline Beecham Vaccines Customer Care Line (0181 913 4116).
- British Airways Travel Clinics (0171 831 5333).
- London School of Tropical Disease (0171 636 8636).
- Department of Communicable and Tropical Diseases, Birmingham (0121 772 3009).
- Department of Infectious Diseases and Tropical Medicine, Manchester (0161 276 8773).
- Liverpool School of Tropical Medicine (0151 708 9393).
- The Communicable Disease Surveillance Centres (CDSC) offer general advice to medical staff on communicable disease surveillance and control (including travel medicine) (see p. 215).
- Malaria prophylaxis — PHLS Malaria Reference Laboratories in London, Birmingham, Oxford, Liverpool and Glasgow (see p. 162, 217).
- The Medical Advisory Service for Travellers Abroad (MASTA) (see p. 215).
- TRAVAX, a constantly updated vaccination service run by the CDSC in Scotland (0141 946 7120, ext. 1277). It includes recommendations for travel immunization and malaria prevention. The system needs a PC, modem and start-up software.
- PRESTEL, p. 50063. Regularly updated by the DoH.

Notes

Travel vaccine administration — summary

Vaccine	Adult dosage	Child dosage	Primary course	Route	Booster
Cholera	0.5 ml (1st) 1 ml (2nd)	1–5 years 0.1 ml (1st) 0.3 ml (2nd) 5–10 years 0.3 ml (1st) 0.5 ml (2nd)	2 doses 4 weeks apart (min. 1 week)	IM/SC (2nd dose may be ID — see booster)	6 months < 10 years 0.1 ml ID > 10 years 0.2 ml ID Adult 0.2 ml ID
Diphtheria	Ads low dose 0.5 ml	< 10 years 0.5 ml Ads Diphth vaccine (consider DTP or DT)	3 doses 4 weeks apart	IM/SC	Preschool (DT) thereafter every 10 years (with Ads low dose vaccine)
Hepatitis A	1 ml (Monodose)	1–15 years 0.5 ml (Junior)	2 doses 2–4 weeks apart (child); 1dose (adults)	IM	Single booster 6–12 months Then 10 years
Hepatitis B	1 ml	0–12 years 0.5 ml	3 doses 0, 1, 6 months Accelerated course: 0, 1, 2 plus 12 months	IM	5–10 years
Japanese B encephalitis	1 ml	< 3 years 0.5 ml > 3 years 1 ml	3 doses 0, 7, 28 days	SC	1–4 years
Meningococcoal: AC VAX;	0.5 ml	> 2 months 0.5 ml	Single dose	SC	> 5 years, 5 years < 5 years, 1–2 years
Meningivac A+C	0.5 ml	> 18 months 0.5 ml	Single dose	IM/SC	3 years

continued

Vaccine	Adult dosage	Child dosage	Primary course	Route	Booster
Poliomyelitis:					
OPV	3 drops or monodose	3 drops or monodose	3 doses 4 weeks apart	Orally	Preschool Leaving school Every 10+ years
IPV	0.5 ml	0.5 ml	3 doses 4 weeks apart	IM/SC	Preschool Leaving school Every 5+ years
Rabies	1 ml	1 ml	3 doses 0, 7, 28 days	IM/SC	2–3 years
Tetanus	0.5 ml	0.5 ml	3 doses 4 weeks apart	IM/SC	Preschool Leaving school Every 10+ years
Tick-borne encephalitis	0.5 ml	0.5 ml	3 doses 2nd: 1–3 months 3rd: 9–12 months	IM	3 years
Tuberculosis (tuberculin negative, except <3 months) ID BCG	0.1 ml	>3 months 0.1 ml <3 months 0.05 ml	Single dose	Strictly ID	None
Typhoid:					
Whole-cell vaccine	0.5 ml 0.1 ml (ID) (2nd)	1–10 years 0.25 ml 0.1 ml (ID) (2nd)	2 doses 4–6 weeks apart	IM/SC 2nd dose may be ID (0.1 ml)	3 years (as 2nd dose)
Vi antigen vaccine	0.5 ml	>18 months 0.5 ml	Single dose	IM/SC	3 years
Oral typhoid vaccine	1 capsule	>6 years 1 capsule	3 doses on alternate days	Orally	3 years; 1 year for frequent travellers
Yellow fever	0.5 ml	>9 months 0.5 ml	Single dose	SC	10 years (for travellers)

Travel from the UK immunization guide

Country	Yellow fever	Cholera	Tuberculosis	Hepatitis A	Hepatitis B	Typhoid	Diphtheria	Tetanus	Polio	Meningococcus A and C	Japanese B encephalitis	Tick-borne encephalitis	Rabies	Malaria prophylaxis
Afghanistan	R		P	R	P	R	P	R	R				R	R
Albania			P	R	P	R	P	R	R			P	P	
Algeria	P		P	R	P	R	P	R	R				P	
Angola	R		P	R	P	R	P	R	R				P	R
Antigua				R		R		R	R					
Argentina (rural and northern)			P	R	P	R	P	R	R				P	R
Australia								R						
Austria								R				P		
Azores								R	R					
Bahamas			R			R		R	R					
Bahrain			P	R	P	R	P	R	R				P	
Bali				R		R		R	R					
Bangladesh			P	R	P	R	P	R	R	P	P		P	R
Barbados				R		R		R	R					
Belgium								R						
Belize		P	P	R	P	R	P	R	R				P	R
Benin Republic	C		P	R	P	R	P	R	R	P			P	R
Bermuda				R		R		R	R					
Bhutan			P	R	P		P	R	R	P	P		P	R
Bolivia	R	P	P	R	P	R	P	R	R				P	R
Botswana			P	R	P	R	P	R	R				P	R
Brazil	R	P	P	R	P	R	P	R	R	P			P	R
Brunei			P	R	P	R	P	R	R			P	P	
Bulgaria			R					R	R				P	
Burkina Faso	C		P	R	P	R	P	R	R	P	P		P	R
Burundi	R		P	R	P	R	P	R	R	P			P	R
Cameroon	C	P	P	R	P	R	P	R	R	R			P	R
Canada								R						
Canary Islands								R						
Cape Verde Islands			P	R	P	R	P	R	R				P	R
Cayman Islands			P	R	P	R	P	R	R					
Central African Republic	C		P	R	P	R	P	R	R	R			P	R

continued

C, compulsory; R, recommended (risk of infection); P, possible risk.

Country	Yellow fever	Cholera	Tuberculosis	Hepatitis A	Hepatitis B	Typhoid	Diphtheria	Tetanus	Polio	Meningococcus A and C	Japanese B encephalitis	Tick-borne encephalitis	Rabies	Malaria prophylaxis
Chad	C		P	R	P	R	P	R	R	R			P	R
Chile		P	P	R	P	R	P	R	R				P	
China			P	R	P	R	P	R	R		P		P	R
Colombia	R	P	P	R	P	R	P	R	R				P	R
Commonwealth of Independent States (formerly USSR)			P	P	P	P	P	R	R			P	P	
Comoros			P	R	P	R	P	R	R				P	
Congo	C		P	R	P	R	P	R	R	R			P	R
Cook Islands			P	R	P	R	P	R	R				P	R
Corsica								R						
Costa Rica		P	P	R	P	R	P	R	R				P	R
Cuba			P	R	P	R	P	R	R					
Cyprus Republic								R						
Czech Republic								R				P		
Denmark								R						
Djibouti		P	P	R	P	R	P	R	R	P			P	R
Dominica			P	R	P	R	P	R	R					
Dominican Republic			P	R	P	R	P	R	R				P	R
Ecuador	R	P	P	R	P	R	P	R	R				P	R
Egypt			P	R	P	R	P	R	R				P	R
El Salvador		P	P	R	P	R	P	R	R				P	R
Ethiopia	R		P	R	P	R	P	R	R	R			P	R
Falkland Islands								R	R					
Fiji			P	R	P	R	P	R	R					
Finland								R				P		
France								R						
French Guiana	C	P	P	R	P	R	P	R	R				P	R
French Polynesia			P	R	P	R	P	R	R					
Gabon	C		P	R	P	R	P	R	R	R			P	R
Gambia	R		P	R	P	R	P	R	R	R			P	R
Germany								R				P		
Ghana	C		P	R	P	R	P	R	R	P			P	R
Gibraltar								R						
Greece (mainland and islands)								R						
Greenland								R						
Grenada			P	R	P	R	P	R	R				P	
Guatemala		P	P	R	P	R	P	R	R				P	R
Guinea Bissau	R	P	P	R	P	R	P	R	R	R			P	R
Guinea Equatorial	R		P	R	P	R	P	R	R	R			P	R
Guinea Republic	R		P	R	P	R	P	R	R	R			P	R
Guyana	R		P	R	P	R	P	R	R				P	R
Haiti			P	R	P	R	P	R	R				P	R

Country	Yellow fever	Cholera	Tuberculosis	Hepatitis A	Hepatitis B	Typhoid	Diphtheria	Tetanus	Polio	Meningococcus A and C	Japanese B encephalitis	Tick-borne encephalitis	Rabies	Malaria prophylaxis
Hawaii								R	R					
Honduras Republic		P	P	R	P	R	P	R	R				P	R
Hong Kong			P	R	P	R	P	R	R		P			
Hungary								R				P		
Ibiza								R						
Iceland								R						
India			P	R	P	R	P	R	R	R	P		P	R
Indonesia			P	R	P	R	P	R	R		P		P	R
Iran			P	R	P	R	P	R	R				P	R
Iraq			P	R	P	R	P	R	R				P	R
Ireland								R						
Israel			P	R	P	R	P	R	R					
Italy								R						
Ivory Coast	C		P	R	P	R	P	R	R	R			P	R
Jamaica			R		R			R	R					
Japan								R			P			
Jordan			P	R	P	R	P	R	R				P	
Kampuchea			P	R	P	R	P	R	R		P		P	R
Kenya	R		P	R	P	R	P	R	R	R			P	R
Korea			P	R	P	R	P	R	R		P		P	
Kuwait			P	R	P	R	P	R	R				P	
Laos			P	R	P	R	P	R	R		P		P	R
Lebanon			P	R	P	R	P	R	R				P	
Lesotho			P	R	P	R	P	R	R				P	
Liberia	C		P	R	P	R	P	R	R	R			P	R
Libya			P	R	P	R	P	R	R				P	
Luxembourg								R						
Madagascar			P	R	P	R	P	R	R				P	R
Madeira								R	R					
Majorca								R	R					
Malawi			P	R	P	R	P	R	R	R			P	R
Malaysia			P	R	P	R	P	R	R		P		P	R
Maldives			P	R	P	R	P	R	R				P	
Mali	C		P	R	P	R	P	R	R	R			P	R
Malta			P					R	R					
Martinique			R		R			R	R					
Mauritania	C		P	R	P	R	P	R	R	P			P	R
Mauritius			P	R	P	R	P	R	R				P	R
Mexico		P	P	R	P	R	P	R	R				P	
Minorca								R	R					
Monaco								R						

continued

C, compulsory; R, recommended (risk of infection); P, possible risk.

TRAVEL IMMUNIZATION GUIDE

Country	Yellow fever	Cholera	Tuberculosis	Hepatitis A	Hepatitis B	Typhoid	Diphtheria	Tetanus	Polio	Meningococcus A and C	Japanese B encephalitis	Tick-borne encephalitis	Rabies	Malaria prophylaxis
Mongolia			P	R	P	R	P	R	R				P	
Morocco			P	R	P	R	P	R	R				P	
Mozambique	C		P	R	P	R	P	R	R	P			P	R
Myanmar (Burma)			P	R	P	R	P	R	R	R	P		P	R
Namibia			P	R	P	R	P	R	R				P	R
Nepal			P	R	P	R	P	R	R	R	P		P	R
Netherlands								R						
Neth. Antilles				R		R		R	R					
New Caledonia			P	R	P	R	P	R	R					
New Zealand								R						
Nicaragua		P	P	R	P	R	P	R	R				P	R
Niger	C		P	R	P	R	P	R	R	R			P	R
Nigeria	R	P	P	R	P	R	P	R	R	R			P	R
Norway								R				P		
Oman			P	R	P	R	P	R	R				P	R
Pakistan			P	R	P	R	P	R	R	P			P	R
Panama	R	P	P	R	P	R	P	R	R					R
Papua New Guinea			P	R	P	R	P	R	R					R
Paraguay			P	R	P	R	P	R	R				P	R
Peru	R	P	P	R	P	R	P	R	R				P	R
Philippines			P	R	P	R	P	R	R	R	P		P	R
Poland								R	R			P		
Portugal								R						
Puerto Rico			P	R	P	R	P	R	R				P	
Quatar			P	R	P	R	P	R	R				P	
Réunion Islands			P		P	R	P	R	R					
Romania			P	P	P	R	P	R	R			P		
Rwanda	C		P	R	P	R	P	R	R	R			P	R
St Lucia			P			R		R	R					
Samoa			P	R	P	R	P	R	R					
Sao Tomé and Principe	C		P	R	P	R	P	R	R	R			P	R
Sardinia								R						
Saudi Arabia			P	R	P	R	P	R	R	R			P	R
Senegal	C		P	R	P	R	P	R	R	R			P	R
Seychelles			P	R	P	R	P	R	R				P	
Sierra Leone	R		P	R	P	R	P	R	R	R			P	R
Singapore			P	R	P	R	P	R	R					
Slovak Republic								R				P		
Solomon Islands			P	R	P	R	P	R	R					R
Somalia	P		P	R	P	R	P	R	R	R			P	R
South Africa			P	R	P	R	P	R	R				P	R
Spain								R						
Sri Lanka			P	R	P	R	P	R	R			P	P	R

Country	Yellow fever	Cholera	Tuberculosis	Hepatitis A	Hepatitis B	Typhoid	Diphtheria	Tetanus	Polio	Meningococcus A and C	Japanese B encephalitis	Tick-borne encephalitis	Rabies	Malaria prophylaxis
Sudan	R		P	R	P	R	P	R	R	R			P	R
Surinam	R		P	P	R	P	P	R	R				P	R
Swaziland			P	R	P	R	P	R	R				P	R
Sweden								R				P		
Switzerland								R				P		
Syria			P	R	P	R	P	R	R				P	R
Taiwan			P	R	P	R	P	R	R		P			
Tanzania	R	P	P	R	P	R	P	R	R	R			P	R
Thailand			P	R	P	R	P	R	R			P	P	R
Tobago				R		R		R	R				P	
Togo	C		P	R	P	R	P	R	R	R			P	R
Trinidad				R		R		R	R				P	
Tunisia			P	R	P	R	P	R	R				P	
Turkey			P	R	P	R	P	R	R				P	R (East)
Uganda	R		P	R	P	R	P	R	R	R			P	R
United Arab Emirates			P	R	P	R	P	R	R				P	R
United States of America								R					P	
Uruguay			P	R	P	R	P	R	R				P	
Vannatu			P	R	P	R	P	R	R					R
Venezuela	R	P	P	R	P	R	P	R	R				P	R
Vietnam			P	R	P	R	P	R	R		P		P	R
Virgin Islands				R		R		R	R					
West Indies				R		R		R	R					
Yemen			P	R	P	R	P	R	R				P	R
Yugoslavia (former)				R		R		R	R			P	P	
Zaire	R		P	R	P	R	P	R	R	R			P	R
Zambia		P	P	R	P	R	P	R	R	R			P	R
Zimbabwe			P	R	P	R	P	R	R	P			P	R

C, compulsory; R, recommended (risk of infection); P, possible risk.
Note: This immunization guide is for short-term travellers arriving at the above countries directly from the UK. It is an information guide and, of course, constantly updated.

Notes

Manufacturers and useful addresses

Air Transport Users Committee (Advice for disabled travellers), Care-in-the-Air,
1229 Kingsway, London WC2B 6NN
Tel: 0171 242 3882

Bayer plc, Strawberry Hill, Newbury, Berks RG13 1JA
Tel: 0635 39000

Bio Products Laboratory, Dagger Lane, Elstree, Herts WR8 0XL
Tel: 0181 905 1818

Blood Transfusion Services, Scotland
Aberdeen: Forester Hill Road, Aberdeen AB9 2ZW
Tel: 01224 681818

Dundee: Ninewells Hospital, Dundee DD1 9SY
Tel: 01382 645166

Glasgow: Law Hospital, Carluke NL8 5ES
Tel: 01698 373315

Edinburgh: Dept of Transfusion Medicine, Royal Infirmary, Laurison Place,
Edinburgh EH3 9HB
Tel: 0131 229 7291

Inverness: Raigmore Hospital, Inverness IV2 3UJ
Tel: 0463 704000

British Airways Travel Clinics
Tel: 0171 831 5333

British Airways Medical Service, Queens Building (N121), Heathrow Airport,
Hounslow, Middlesex
Tel: 0181 526 7070

British Diabetic Association, 10 Queen Anne Street, London W1M 0BD
Tel: 0171 323 1531

Cambridge Laboratories, Cambridge Selfcare Diagnostic Ltd, Richmond House, Old
Brewery Road, Sandyford Lane, Newcastle upon Tyne NE2 1XG
Tel: 0191 261 5950

Committee on the Safety of Medicines, 1 Nine Elms Lane, London SW8 5NQ
Tel: 0171 273 3000

Communicable Disease Surveillance Centres
London: 61 Collingdale Avenue, London NW9 5HT
Tel: 0181 200 6868

Wales: Abton House, Wetal Road, Roath, Cardiff CF4 3QX
Tel: 01222 521997

Scotland: Ruchill Hospital, Bilsland Drive, Glasgow G20 9NB
Tel: 0141 946 7120 (ext: 1277 for Travax service)

Department of Communicable & Tropical Diseases, Birmingham Heartlands
  Hospital, Bordesley Green East, Birmingham B9 5ST
    Tel: 0121 766 6611
Department of Infectious Diseases and Tropical Medicine in Manchester (Travel
  Clinic)
    Tel: 0161 276 8773
Department of Health, Richmond House, 79 Whitehall, London SW1A 2NS
    Tel: 0171 210 3000
Duphar Laboratories Ltd, Gaters Hill, West End, Southampton SO3 3JD
    Tel: 01703 472281
Evans Medical Ltd, Evans House, Regent Park, Kingston Road, Leatherhead, Surrey
  KT22 7PQ
    Tel: 01372 364000 (vaccine orders)
    Tel: 01372 364100 (medical information), 01625 537607 (24-h advice line)
Farillon Ltd, Ashton Road, Romford, Essex RM3 6WE
    Tel: 01708 379000
Geer Laboratories, Inc., PO Box 800, Lenoir, NC 28645, USA
    Tel: 001 704 754 5327
Homeway Ltd, The White House, Littleton, Winchester, Hants SO22 6QS
    Tel: 01962 881526
Hospital for Tropical Disease, 4 St Pancras Way, London NW1
    Tel: 0171 387 4411
Immuno Ltd, Rye Lane, Dunton Green, Sevenoaks, Kent TN14 5HB
    Tel: 01732 458101
John Radcliffe Hospital, Headley Way, Oxford OX3 9DU
    Tel: 01865 741166
The Laboratories, Belfast City Hospital, Lisburn Road, Belfast BT9 7AB
    Tel: 01232 329241
Lederle Laboratories, Fareham Road, Gosport, Hants PO13 0AS
    Tel: 01329 22400
Liverpool School of Tropical Medicine, Pembroke Place, Liverpool L3 5QA
    Tel: 0151 708 9393
London School of Hygiene & Tropical Medicine, Keppel Street, London WC1E 7HT
    Tel: 0171 636 8636
Manchester Monsall Hospital, Monsall Road, Manchester M10 8WR
    Tel: 0161 795 4567
Medical Advisory Service for Travellers Abroad, London School of Hygiene and
  Tropical Medicine, Keppel Street, London WC1E 7HT
    Tel: 0171 631 4408
    Tel: 0891 224 100 (24-h advice, payline)
Merck, Sharp & Dohme Ltd, Hertford Road, Hoddesdon, Herts EN11 9BU
    Tel: 01992 467272
Merieux UK Ltd, Clivemont Road, Maidenhead, Berks SL6 7BU
    Tel: 01628 785291; 01628 773737 (Vaccination Information Service)
Pharmacia, Davy Avenue, Knowhill, Milton Keynes MK5 8PH
    Tel: 01908 661101
Prescription Pricing Authority
    Tel: 0191 232 5371
Public Health Laboratory Services, 61 Collingdale Avenue, London, NW9 5HT
    Tel: 0181 200 6868

PHLS Malaria Reference Laboratories
Birmingham: Birmingham Heartlands Hospital, Bordesley Green East, Birmingham B9 5ST
   Tel: 0121 766 6611
Oxford: Churchill Hospital, Oxford OX3 7LJ
   Tel: 01865 225570
Liverpool: Liverpool School of Tropical Medicine, Pembroke Place, Liverpool L3 5QA
   Tel: 0151 708 9393
Glasgow: Ruchill Hospital, Bilsland Drive, Glasgow G20 9NB
   Tel: 0141 946 7120
London: London School of Hygiene & Tropical Medicine, Keppel Street, London WC1E 7HT
   Tel: 0171 636 8636, 0171 636 3924. For clinical advice — Tel: 0171 387 4411; advice to the public on maleria — Tel: 0891 600 350; recorded advice — Tel: 0171 636 7921
Meningococcal vaccine advice
   Tel: 0161 445 2416 (Manchester), 0141 946 7120 (Scotland), 0181 200 6868 (London)

Regent Labs Ltd, 861 Coronation Road, Park Royal, London NW10 7PT
   Tel: 0181 961 6868
Regional Virus Laboratory, Royal Victoria Hospital, Grosvenor Road, Belfast BT12 6BA
   Tel: 01232 240503
Royal Association for Disability and Rehabilitation, 12 City Forum, 250 City Road, London EC1V 8OS
   Tel: 0171 250 3222
Servier Laboratories Ltd, Fulmer Hall, Windmill Road, Fulmer, Slough SL3 6HH
   Tel: 01753 662744
SmithKline Beecham Pharmaceuticals, Mundells, Welwyn Garden City, Herts AL7 1EY
   Tel: 01707 325111, 0181 9134116 (customer care line)
Tripscope, Pamwell House, 160 Pennywell Road, Bristol BSS 0TX
   Tel: 0117 9414 094
Yellow Fever Vaccination Centres, Department of Health, Room 554, Richmond House, 79 Whitehall, London SW1A 2NS
   Tel: 0171 210 5039

Index